THE
TUBBY TRAVELER
FROM
TOPEKA

Bros S. Edward

THE
TUBBY TRAVELER
FROM
TOPEKA

A Unique Case Study of a Bon Vivant's Travels Around the World

BRIAN S. EDWARDS MD

The Tubby Approach to Diet and Exercise

The Bridge between the Tubby Factor
and Low-Carbohydrate Diets

Library of Congress Control Number:		2012903904
ISBN:	Hardcover	978-1-4691-7746-5
	Softcover	978-1-4691-7745-8
	Ebook	978-1-4691-7747-2

This book was printed in the United States of America.

To order additional copies of this book, contact:
Xlibris Corporation
1-888-795-4274
www.Xlibris.com
Orders@Xlibris.com
108257

Note To Readers

This book is owned by Lipid King LLC.

This book reflects my opinions which I have tried to substantiate with numerous references.

I thank the many people who have taught me what I know from the National Lipid Association and the Obesity Society.

In particular I rely very heavily on the writings of Gary Taube, Dr. Aronne, Dr Atkins, Dr. Bray, Gina Kolata, the Medical Clinics of North America Sept. 2011 edition on Obesity.

I have tried to give credit to many sources. If I missed some quotation marks I am truly sorry. My main original contribution is The Sponge Syndrome. Other than this I have tried to give credit to the many textbooks from 2011 that reflect the sea change or paradigm shift in thought.

In particular I want to thank Dr. Gardner and Dr. Sachs for their trials whose findings I repeat many times in this book.

This all started with a talk at a NLA meeting in Washington DC. when Dr. D. Mozaffarian gave a talk about dietary fats on August 27, 2010.

Finally, the reader should consult their physician before they adopt the suggestions I make in this book.

Other books by Dr. Edwards:

The Tubby Theory From Topeka
The Fen-Fen Diet Pill Program

Contents

Prefix 1 9

Prefix 2 10

Prefix 3 13

Prefix 4 18

Prefix 5 20

Prefix 6 21

Prefix 7 24

Prefix 8 27

PART 1

Twelve Months of Travel on a Low-Carb Diet

Chapter 1   Scotland and Ireland...31

Chapter 2   Florida...39

Chapter 3   Mardi Gras and Texas...43

Chapter 4   Hong Kong to Athens Cruise 49

Chapter 5   Barhopping in New York City 53

Chapter 6   Hawaii..57

Chapter 7   European River Cruise 61

Chapter 8   Paradise Island, Atlantis, Bahamas 65

Chapter 9   Alaskan Cruise...69

Chapter 10 Orlando 75

Chapter 11 Palm Desert, California..81

Chapter 12 Paul Gauguin Cruise to Society Islands and Marquesas.....85

PART II

Adjusting to sea change in science.

Chapter 13 Introduction to Part II..131

Chapter 14 The Tubby Approach to Diet and Exercise 135

Chapter 15 Weight Loss and Exercise: A False Hope 139

Chapter 16 Obesity Core Conference 10-1-2011.................................149

Chapter 17 The History of Obesity and Diets 231
Chapter 18 Old Game Plan 239
Chapter 19 The Reduced Obese 243
Chapter 20 The Great Fat Debate 247
Chapter 21 Caveat emptor: 253
Chapter 22 Gardner and Sachs Trial 257
Chapter 23 The Look-AHEAD Trial 263
Chapter 24 Calories In, Calories Out? 265
Chapter 25 Healthy Diet 271
Chapter 26 How Does a Low-Carbohydrate Diet Work? 275
Chapter 27 Victoza (Liraglutide) May Be the New Miracle Drug 279
Chapter 28 Cancer Update 283
Chapter 29 Twiggies May Also Have Metabolic Syndrome 289
Chapter 30 Update on the Tubby Theory from Topeka 295
Chapter 31 Epilogue 298

Bibliography 303
Index 307

Prefix I

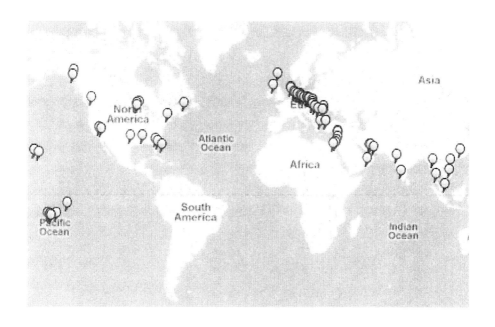

Prefix 2

Summary List of Travels 2011

1.	Aviemore and the Cairngorms, Scotland	1-15-11 to 1-23-11
2.	Dublin, Ireland	1-22-11 to 1-26-11
3.	Athlone, Ireland	1-27-11 to 2-1-11
4.	Wyndham Bonnet Creek Resort, Florida	2-13-11 to 2-19-11
4a.	Jensen Beach, Henderson Island, Florida	2-19-11 to 3-5-11
4b.	W New Orleans Hotel, Louisiana	3-6-11 to 3-11-11
4c.	Hyatt Regency Lost Pines Resort and Spa, Texas	3-11-11 to 3-13-11
4d.	Westin Mission Hills Villas	3-19-11 to 3-24-11
5.	Oceania Cruise on the Nautica	3-26-11 to 5-10-11
6.	Hue, Thua Thien, Hue Province, Vietnam	3-29-11
7.	Ho Chi Minh City, Vietnam	4-1-11 to 4-2-11
8.	Singapore	4-3-11
9.	Phuket, Thailand	4-5-11
10.	Yangon (Rangoon), Myanmar	1-7-11 to 1-9-11
11.	Kochi, Kerala, India	4-13-11
12.	Mumbai (Bombay), Maharashtra, India	4-13-11
13.	Muscat, Oman	4-18-11
14.	Dubai, United Arab Emirates	4-19-11 to 4-20-11

15.	Fujairah, United Arab Emirates	4-22-11
16.	Port Sultan Qaboos, Oman	4-23-11
17.	Salalah, Oman	4-25-11
18.	Gulf of Amen and Red Sea	4-26-11 to 4-29-11
19.	Aqaba, Jordan	4-30-11
20.	Luxor, Nile River Valley, Egypt	5-1-11 to 5-2-11
21.	Safaga, Red Sea, and Sinai	5-1-11 to 5-2-11
22.	Sharm El Sheikh, South Sinai, Egypt	
23.	Suez Canal, Egypt	5-4-11
24.	Jerusalem, Israel	5-5-11 to 5-6-11
25.	Haifa, Israel	5-7-11
26.	Ephesus, Izmir Province, Egypt (Kusadasi)	5-9-11
27.	Athens, Greece	5-10-11 to 5-13-11
28.	Sheraton New York Hotel and Towers	5-18-11 to 5-23-11
29.	Ka'anapali Beach Club, Maui, Hawaii	5-29-11 to 6-10-11
30.	St. Regis Princeville Resort, Princeville, Kauai	6-10-11 to 6-12-11
31.	The Point at Poipu, Kauai, Hawaii	6-12-11 to 6-25-11
32.	Hotel Pulitzer, Amsterdam, Noord-Holland, the Netherlands	6-30-11 to 7-2-11
33.	Kinderdijk, Zuid-Holland, the Netherlands	7-3-11
34.	Cologne, North Rhine-Westphalia	7-4-11
35.	Kobenz, Rhineland-Palatinate	7-5-11
36.	Miltenburg, Germany	7-6-11
37.	Wurzburg, Romantic Road, Germany	7-7-11
38.	Bamberg, Bavaria, Germany	7-8-11
39.	Nuremburg, Germany	7-9-11
40.	Regensburg, Bavaria, Germany	7-10-11
41.	Passau, Bayerischer Wald, Germany	7-11-11
42.	Melk, Danube Valley, Austria	7-12-11
43.	Durnstein, Danube Valley	7-12-11
44.	Vienna, Austria	7-13-11
45.	Bratislavia, Slovakia	7-14-11
46.	Budapest, Hungary	7-15-11 to 7-16-11
47.	Kalocza, Hungary	7-17-11
48.	Vukovar, Croatia	7-18-11

49.	Osijek, Croatia	7-18-11
50.	Belgrade, Serbia	7-19-11
51.	Iron Gate on the Danube River	7-20-11
52.	Viminacium, Serbia	7-20-11
53.	Veliko, Turnovo, Serbia	7-21-11
53.	Arbanasi, Serbia	7-21-11
54.	Belogradchik Fortress	7-22-11
55.	Bucharest, Romania	7-23-11
56.	Jensen Beach	7-7-11 to 7-11-11
57.	Harborside Resort, Atlantis, Nassau	7-11-13 to 7-20-11
58.	Westin Seattle, Washington	8-31-11 to 9-3-11
59.	Holland-American Cruise to Alaska	9-3-11 to 9-10-11
60.	Juneau, Alaska	
61.	Sitka, Alaska	
62.	Kitchacan, Alaska	
63.	Tracy Arm Glacier	
64.	Victoria, Canada	9-9-11
65.	Orlando, Florida	9-30-11 to 10-5-11
	Mall of Amercian, Minneapolis	
66.	Itazys Resort, Viz Onamia, Minnesota	10-8-11 to 10-15-11
	Duluth, Minnesota	
67.	Westin Mission Hills, Rancho Mirage, California	11-11-11 to 11-14-11
68.	SLS Hotel LA, California	11-15-11 to 11-19-11
69.	Gaughin Cruise Tahiti	11-19-11 to 12-3-11
70.	Papeete	
71.	Fakarava	
72.	Fatu Hiva, Manavave, Marquesas	
73.	Hiva Oa	
74.	Huku Hiva	
75.	Taha	
76.	Bora-Bora	
78.	Moorea	
79.	Jensen Beach	

12-19-11 to 1-5-12

Prefix 3

Lipidology Glossary

The Blood Tests

1. LDL-C: The C stands for cholesterol. This is the bad cholesterol. It is determined from a blood test. It is a calculated number and is often discordant with the newer, better test, LDL-P. The P stands for particle.
2. LDL-P: The number of particles (P) that carry the cholesterol is the best predictor of cardiovascular risk. It is determined by a blood test and an NMR machine. ApoB is another way to measure the atherogenic particles. High-fat diets make large LDL-P, while low-fat diets make for more small, dense LDL-P. There is much confusion about size being important for risk stratification. The National Lipid Association meetings preach that size doesn't matter most of the time. No double entendre intended.
3. HDL-C: This has been called the good cholesterol. Ratios are often used to determine cardiovascular risk. The AIM-HIGH trial and the fact that there are proinflammatory or bad HDL-Cs make the ratio with HDL-C less reliable. Low-fat diets lower HDL-C. High-fat diets raise HDL-C.
4. HDL-P: The particle number will rise with the HDL-C till about a level of 60 dl/ml on the HDL-C. At this point, as the HDL-C goes higher, the size of the HDL-P gets larger. What does it all mean? It's a conundrum as the critical test is the functionality of the HDL-P. There is no clinical lab test for functionality at this time.
5. Triglycerides: Three fatty acids make up a triglyceride. Low-carbohydrate diets have low triglycerides. Low-fat diets have high triglycerides.

6. Tubby Factor: I coined this term as the technical term non-HDL cholesterol was too confusing. This is the second-best predictor of cardiovascular risk. It is all the cholesterol without the HDL-C. Take the "total cholesterol" level on your lipid panel and subtract the HDL-C. This is also often discordant with the LDL-C especially in people with metabolic syndrome.

Medical Imaging

7. CAC (coronary calcium score): This is a CT scan of the heart. It can show if a patient has plaque in his coronary arteries. No IV, no dye involved.
8. CIMT (carotid intima-medial wall thickness): Ultrasound of the carotid arteries in the neck that measures the thickness of the wall of the carotid. It is different from the duplex carotid ultrasound that measures the flow of the blood in the carotid and determines how much blockage there is in the carotid.

Diabetic Terms

9. Metabolic syndrome: This is a prediabetic state with apple obesity, high blood pressure, high triglycerides, and low HDL-C.
10. Hgb A1C: Hemoglobin A1C is a blood test to determine the average glucose level in the blood over the last one or two months.
11. Prediabetes: A fasting glucose 100 or greater.
12. Apple obesity: A waist greater than forty inches in males or thirty-five inches in females.
13. High blood pressure: Greater than 130 systolic.
14. High triglycerides: Greater than 150.
15. Low HDL-C: Lower than forty for males and lower than fifty for females.

Reduced obese

A person who has lost a significant amount of weight and now has a different metabolism from obese people and normal-weight people. The reduced obese now has a body that is using several compensatory mechanisms to gain weight.

Set Point

Metab Syndr Relat Disord, 2011 Apr. 9, (2):85-9. Epub 2010 Nov. 30.
Set-Point Theory and Obesity
Farias, M. M.; Cuevas, A. M.; Rodriguez, F.
Source:
Department of Nutrition and Metabolism, Pontificia Universidad Catolica de
Chile, Santiago, Chile.

Abstract from the above article.

"Obesity is a consequence of the complex interplay between genetics and environment. Several studies have shown that body weight is maintained at a stable range, known as the 'set-point,' despite the variability in energy intake and expenditure. Additionally, it has been shown that the body is more efficient protecting against weight loss during caloric deprivation compared to conditions of weight gain with overfeeding, suggesting an adaptive role of protection during periods of low food intake. Emerging evidence on bariatric surgery outcomes, particularly gastric bypass, suggests a novel role of these surgical procedures in establishing a new set-point by alterations in body weight regulatory physiology, therefore resulting in sustainable weight loss results. Continuing research is necessary to elucidate the biological mechanisms responsible for this change, which may offer new options for the global burden of obesity."

Plateau: After 8% or more weight loss, it becomes difficult to lose more weight.

Resettlement point: New term for plateau. Obese people have high levels of leptin. Some believe there is a resistance to leptin as you get obese. Insulin levels also get higher in the obese due to insulin resistance. Others believe the obese have a high leptin threshold. Fat cells make leptin. As the fat cells shrink, less leptin is made. If the threshold is high in the obese and the leptin level goes below a threshold that alerts the brain that the body is starving, the body starts compensatory mechanisms to gain the weight back. The threshold level of leptin changes in the obese, making it difficult to maintain weight loss.

Energy gap: "These formulas would predict an energy gap of 190-200 kcal/day for a 100 kg person losing 10% of body weight and an energy gap of 280-300 kcal/day for this same person losing 15% of body weight (Figure 4). The energy gap for weight loss maintenance can provide an estimate of how much behavior change is required to maintain a given amount of weight loss. This analysis indicates that in order to create and maintain significant body weight loss (i.e., obesity treatment) large behavioral changes are needed. This is in stark contrast to primary obesity prevention in which small behavioral changes can eliminate the small energy imbalance that occurs before the body has gained significant weight. Because the body has not previously stored this 'new' excess energy, it does not defend against the behavioral strategies as happens when the body loses weight."

J Am Diet Assoc. Author manuscript; available in PMC 2010 November 1.

Published in final edited form as:

J Am Diet Assoc. 2009 November; 109(11): 1848-1853. doi: 10.1016/j.jada. 2009.08.007

PMCID: PMC2796109

NIHMSID: NIHMS155611

Using the Energy Gap to Address Obesity: A Commentary

James O. Hill, PhD, Professor of Pediatrics and Medicine, Director, John C. Peters, PhD, Associate Director, and Holly R. Wyatt, MD, Associate Professor

Leptin threshold: "Dieting means less fat in your body's fat cells, and it also means a lower level of leptin. When you go below your personal leptin threshold, your brain thinks you're starving. The body has ways of handling this apparent crisis, initiating a number of processes designed to keep you from starving, and raise the level of leptin back up above your personal leptin threshold. Unfortunately these processes can also sabotage your diet" (Jody Smith, June 2010).

Leptin resistance: "Although leptin is a circulating signal that reduces appetite, obese individuals generally exhibit an unusually high circulating concentration of leptin.[56] These people are said to be resistant to the effects of leptin, in much the same way that people with type 2 diabetes are resistant to the effects of insulin. The high sustained concentrations of leptin from the enlarged adipose stores result in leptin desensitization. The pathway of leptin control in obese people might be flawed at some point so the body does not adequately receive the satiety feeling subsequent to eating" (Wikipedia).

Sponge Syndrome: I coined this term because the definitions above are very complicated and not yet fully understood. I know from personal experience that after losing 80 lbs., I gained 58 lbs. despite two to three hours of exercise a day over a forty-three-month period. I gained 1.35 lbs. a month. I gained weight like a sponge due to my body's energy gap, which develops after losing weight, and this energy gap gets larger as the amount of weight loss gets larger.

Moral hazard of obesity: Once someone is obese, there is a general belief that weight loss should only be obtained through deprivation and exercise. If someone is fat, it is their fault.

The theory that weight loss can be maintained with a high-fat diet and little exercise has been felt to be impossible.

Calorie (cal.) and kilocalorie (kcal) are used interchangeably in this book.

Prefix 4

Five Rules of the Tubby Approach to Diet and Exercise

1. Avoid carbohydrates (< 20 g, < 40 g, < 80 g).
2. Don't worry about fat intake. If it tastes good, eat it.
3. Have 30 g of protein with each meal, at least three meals a day.
4. Walk twenty to forty minutes a day. If diabetic, the more exercise the better.
5. Follow your fasting blood glucose and LDL-P three times a year.

The Tubby Theory from Topeka
Five Steps to Prevent Heart Attacks and Strokes and Sudden Death

1. Calculate Tubby Factor (non-HDL cholesterol).
2. CAC (coronary artery calcium obtained with CT scan).
3. CIMT (carotid intimal thickness obtained with ultrasound of the neck).
4. Combination therapy with generic statin (lipitor now generic) and Endur-acin (over-the-counter niacin).
5. Repeat CIMT every two to three years.

To start out, do what is easy. I have tried to outline the easiest program. These are very cost-efficient.

Don't worry about losing weight, but weigh yourself every morning before eating. Don't worry about a three pound weight change. Have a plan to exercise a little more and eat a little less if you gain more than 3 lbs.

Compliance is what it is all about. Outcomes are what it is all about. If people can't follow the instructions, the program does no good. If people are told that if the food tastes good, spit it out, the program will not last long.

I know people love their bread, pasta, and dessert, but once you adapt to high fat and high protein, you will be satisfied and not hungry. It takes one to two months to adapt to the low-carbohydrate diet. Eat all the protein and fat you want till you are full. Tubbies don't know what full means, but as long as you don't eat more than 20 g of carbs a day, I don't think you will gain weight (if you are not completely sedentary as in driving a car for twelve hours a day). Low-calorie diets do not work after two to five years. Why suggest them?

Prefix 5

Bon Vivant

Noun bon vivant (plural bons vivants): A person who enjoys the good things in life, especially good food and drink; a man about town.

This book is a unique case study of a bon vivant going on six cruises in the year 2011 with almost ninety days of cruise cuisine. I show that twelve months of eating 60% fat did not elevate my cholesterol level (LDL-P) significantly nor did it increase the atheroma in the wall of my carotid on CIMT. I found that a low-carbohydrate diet did satiate my appetite. This is the most important concept.

I knew I did not want to go back to the world of substarvation. I was retired at fifty-eight years old, and I was disappointed that I had gained back 58 lbs. after losing 80 lbs. on a traditional low-calorie diet. I was disappointed again when I gained the weight back after almost five years of exercising two to three hours a day. I suffered from the Sponge Sam syndrome.

In January 2011, I wanted to enjoy life to the fullest and thus embarked on a fabulous year of traveling, eating, and drinking. There must be a moral hazard to this type of "high fat with alcohol" living. My lab work shows in my case study that there was not a price to pay for the high fat. I might not have lost weight on my low-carb diet, but at least I did not continue to gain weight as I had the previous four years on a "healthy" diet with hours of exercise.

Prefix 6

The Sponge Syndrome in the Reduced Obese

I heard a commentator say that despite all its faults, Herman Cain's message of 999 has been heard throughout the USA. People may not know exactly what it is, but it has brought the tax code to their attention. I hate to say it, but lipidology is about as exciting at the tax code to the common man. I heard the tax code has 72,000 pages. The lipid literature far exceeds that.

The phrase "reduced obese" is an example of a term that has not caught on in the teachings of obesity. No weight-reduction diet should be considered without referral to this concept. The term has been around for a while, and I only learned of it recently. We have set point, plateau, leptin resistance, leptin threshold, and resettlement point. Any PhD out there confused yet? I call it the Sponge Syndrome. People who lose significant weight get the Sponge Syndrome. They soak up weight like a sponge.

The Reduced Obese

I heard of the term reduced obese for the first time at the Obesity Society meeting in Orlando.

The science of obesity has exploded. The problem is extremely complex. It's all about treating the reduced obese or weight loss maintenance. No one knows the answers. The FDA has shot down the last four diet pills. Combination diet pills will be the answer in the future. The problem is that 60% of the U.S. population will need the pills. That means many pregnant women may take it by accident. The last diet pill had to pay out $2 billion in damages. In the meantime, it is bariatric surgery that is saving lives. It saves lives; but too many people are getting the surgery, and the long term data is not in yet.

The Reduced Obese

This is the problem. It's not what the best diet is. It's not low-fat versus low-carb diet. It is how you do not regain weight once you lost it. There is no solution right now. In the future there will be combination medication and prevention with genetic and phenotype screening for babies. Prevention is the solution, but we do not have a clue about how to do this right now.

I am a one of the reduced obese. In my particular case, I have stopped gaining weight by going on a very low-carbohydrate diet. If you are tubby or have the metabolic syndrome, which means you are insulin resistant, you should try to stay on a low-carb diet. However, there are clearly obese people who do not respond to low-carbohydrate diets. These people are probably not insulin resistant and perhaps have a CC genotype.

It gets worse. An insulin-resistant patient may have lost weight with a low-carb diet, but then when he loses 50 lbs., he may no longer be insulin resistant, and the low-carb diet may not work as well. More importantly, the patient who loses > 8% body weight falls off the obese EE (energy expenditure) slope. It's as if a virus has jumped species. He has hit his settling point or plateau, and the leptin plateau is reached. He becomes hungry, slows metabolism, and anabolism of fat occurs.

It's as if you are winning at poker and suddenly you find yourself playing blackjack. That is what falling off the energy expenditure slope you lost weight with to an EE slope that is more efficient means. The key to all this is satiety. I found satiety with 30 g of protein with three meals a day, high-fat and low-carbohydrate diet. This gives me the time and space to learn to not overeat.

It is not about hypocalorie diets and exercise. The Look AHEAD trial showed 6% weight loss after four years. The results look good till you see the graph's upward trend. This study screened 50,000 people and found 5,000 of the most motivated people. Behavior therapy does not work because the people develop Sponge Syndrome. It may take five to ten years but most of the weight is regained despite all the tips to correct eating behaviors. Diet and exercise programs have and will fail because of the reduced obese problem.

Look at the people who have succeeded at maintaining weight loss. The National Weight Control Registry (NWCR) has a list of 6,000 people who have succeeded. God bless them and God have mercy on them. In the "Obesity" issue of *Medical Clinics of North America* dated September 2011, on page 945, Dubnov-Raz and Berry write, "Both men and women (in the NWCR) consumed a low-fat diet (24%) and exercised to use 470 to 360 calories kcal/d, respectively. The net energy balance was 918 kcal/d for women and 1,225 kcal/d for men. These reduced obese subjects ate an average of five meals a day and conducted a very regimented existence." Every commercial diet program must have a disclaimer at the bottom of their advertisement.

If this product is successful, you will become one of the reduced obese. The adverse effects of this condition:

1. The leptin threshold (plateau or settling point) will be reached.
2. This will make you hungrier, decrease your metabolism, and cause your body to make fat faster and easier.
3. It will take you off your high calorie expending physiology (EE) and knock you over to a new energy expending physiology that will force you to be on a very low-calorie, high-exercise product as achieved by the 6,000 people in the National Weight Control Registry. It has been said that if you maintain the strict diet and exercise for five years, you will finally lose the excess adipocytes and go back to a normal EE (energy expenditure curve). Since the people in the National Weight Control Registry continue to maintain their weight loss by staying on a diet that is 7 cal/lb. and walk 5 miles a day, it seems that successful reduced obese do not return to a normal EE (expenditure physiology).
4. To be on a substarvation diet forever (7 cal/lb.) may scar your psyche similar to concentration camp internees (see Ancel Keys study).

I was walking around the Mall of America and spotted a Square Pants Sponge Bob statue. I thought that was a good way to describe why the reduced obese gain weight. People who have lost 10% of their weight eventually develop the Sponge Syndrome. They soak up calories like a sponge. The concept of the reduced obese has not been taught or accepted into the paradigm of obesity. We continue to blame the obese for their weight as simply calories in versus calories out. Similar to the problem of teaching non-HDL cholesterol, the reduced obese is a terrible term. I propose we associate the concept of the reduced obese as the Sponge Syndrome. I proposed in my prior book that we teach the concept of non-HDL cholesterol as the Tubby Factor.

Prefix 7

The Bizzaro Mathematics of Obesity on the Plateau Planet of the Tubbies

Matrices: (AXB) — (BXA) is not always zero. See chapter 27.

The math of the reduced obese (Tubbies who have lost weight and have hit the plateau) changes because of leptin, insulin, ghrelin, and GLP and falling off the normal EE (energy expenditure) curve to a slower metabolism. It is not simply calories in and calories out once an obese person loses more than 10% body weight. Diet and exercise are not the cure for obesity. As a nutritionist said to me at a recent National Lipidology conference, "Just don't get fat in the first place." The change of weight in humans is multifactoral.

1. Calories in and energy expended is the golden mathematical rule in the twiggy (nonobese) world.

2. Calories are discounted in the plateau world of the Tubbies (obese).

3. Genetics play a major role. Racial differences between China and Western Europe are obvious.

4. Hormones play a major role. Carbohydrates drive insulin, which drives fat accumulation. In the tubby plateau world, people are largely insulin resistant. This means the obese use more insulin to keep the glucose level normal. More insulin causes more hunger and causes the apple-shaped obesity.

5.   Apple obesity fat secretes adipokines. They are inflammatory chemicals that change the biology of the Tubbies (obese).

6.   The biodome of the human intestine contains 800 different types of bacteria. Tubbies (obese) have different bacteria than Twiggies (thin folks), which may account for a difference of absorption of calories.

7.   Finally, some calories are good for the obese (fat and protein) and some are bad (carbohydrates).

The Reduced Obese (Tubbies)

They have a different calorie math, different intestines, different brains, and a weak insulin molecule. This can explain why twiggy calorie mathematics doesn't work for them. A golden rule in skinny math: walking 1 mile = 100 calories. Corollaries to this rule are that running only burns a few more calories. More weight on the body burns a few more calories.

Okay, let's say our thin man walks 4 miles a day. That is roughly 400 calories a day. Twiggy world math is easy:

2,000 calories for resting metabolism
400 calories for walking
Total calories expended: 2,400 calories
This thin man has to eat 2,400 calories a day to maintain his weight. If he stops drinking a can of soda each day (which is about 700 calories a week), he will lose a pound a month.

The bizarro plateau world of the obese has a different mathematics. The bizarro rule of exercise metabolism after losing 10% body weight is that the body's metabolism burns 42% less calories during exercise.

Thus, the obese who have lost 10% of their weight will start to hit the plateau, and when they walk 4 miles, they will not burn 100 calories. They will burn about 60 calories per mile.

More plateau math rules:

1.   If the same exercise is done every day, the muscle memory will burn 10% less calories.
2.   As we age, our resting metabolism decreases 2% each decade.

3. The resting metabolism is not 10 calories per pound. It is probably 7 calories per pound.

I lost 80 lbs. in 2006 by a traditional low-calorie diet called "The Three-Hour Diet" by Jorge Cruise. I decreased my intake to 1,850 calories and then to 1,650 calories and then to 1,450 calories. I exercised one to two hours a day. I ate every three hours. I included carbs at breakfast and lunch but avoided them at dinnertime. When I hit 200 lbs., I was cold all the time. I could not lose any more weight. I became one of the reduced obese. I developed the Sponge Syndrome.

I slowly gained back 50 lbs. in 3.5 years as I increased my diet from 1,500 to 3,000 calories a day. I was told if I exercised ninety minutes a day, I would maintain my weight loss. I exercised at least two hours a day and up to three hours when I hired two different physical trainers. I still continued to gain weight on the average of 1.5 lbs. per month. I did not realize that I have to maintain a diet of 1800 calories a day for the rest of my life to maintain my weight loss.

Next time your doctor tells you to lose weight with diet and exercise, ask him what he advises you do once you become one of the reduced obese and then have to continue a low-calorie diet with more exercise just to maintain the weight loss. Only 6,000 dieters have been documented to maintain their weight loss for five years. To lose 10% of your weight dooms you to a life of restraint that is unsustainable except for a few. If your doctor tells you it's only a matter of discipline and willpower, ask him how to maintain a substarvation diet with 5 miles of walking a day during illness, family holidays, injury, job loss, or stress. The reduced obese are also besieged by compensatory physiological mechanisms in their brain that heighten hunger. These compensatory mechanisms to prevent starvation are what cause the Sponge Syndrome.

Ask your doctor why he is advising a plan that is doomed to fail after five years in 95% of people.

Prefix 8

Summary of Five Low-Carb Diet Studies

"In summary, despite several beneficial properties of Low Carbohydrate over Low Fat diets, even the high quality studies continue to generate conflicting results" (Dubnov-Raz and Berry, p. 943).

Caveat emptor:

"This article focuses on the larger longer term, randomized trials . . . Four studies comparing various diet regimens for weight loss are of particular interest."

1. Dansinger: 60% completed diet . . . no statistical difference between diets. One year, 160 participants. JAMA 2005; 293(1):43-53,

2. Truby: 10% weight loss in all diets after one year, 293 participants. BMJ 2006; 332:1309-14

3. Gardner: Lipid profile and blood pressure changes were better in the Atkins group. 80% completed diets. 311 participants. JAMA; 2007; 297(9): 969-77.

4. Shai: 322 employees, 85% completed program, two-year program.
    a. Low-carbohydrate and Mediterranean diets had greater weight loss than low-fat.
    b. Lipid profile improved the best in the low-carbohydrate diet.

   c. The inflammatory marker increased CRP decreased by more than 20% only in the low-carbohydrate diet and Mediterranean diet.

   d. Only the Mediterranean diet decreased plasma glucose levels in a subgroup of diabetics.

N Engl J Med 2008; 359:229-41
Dubnov-Raz and Berry pp. 941-942
Obesity
LeRoith and Karnieli
Medical Clinics of North America
September 2011, volume 95, number 5

5. Sachs: "The largest and most clear-cut of these head to head trials lasted 2 years with 811 patients and 80% completion rate . . . There was no difference between diets," N Engl J Med. 360(9): 859-873.

Quote from p. 191, *A Guide to Obesity and Metabolic Syndrome: Origins and Treatment* by George Bray. CRC Press 2011.

There was time that low carbohydrate was considered a fad diet and dangerous because of its high fat content. It amazes that the experts underplay the profound surprise that these five major trials brought to the low-fat diet enthusiasts. This is a sea change!

PART 1

Twelve Months of Travel on a Low-Carb Diet

Tubby Thought

"Benefits of Very Little Exercise Demonstrated in Medical Studies

Activity Benefit

55 flights of stairs a week	33% lower death rate
One hour of gardening a week	66% lower risk of sudden cardiac death
Walking one hour a week	51% lower risk of coronary disease
Exercising 30 minutes just 6 days a month	43% lower mortality
Regular demanding household cleaning	Lowered heart attack risk by 54% in men and more than 84% in women"

"Researchers reviewed 44 exercise studies and found that most of the benefits of exercise kick in with the first 1,000 Calories of increased activity each week . . . To burn 1,000 calories a week, or about 145 Calories a day, most people need to increase their activity slightly."

From *Introduction to Clinical Nutrition*, 2012, 3rd edition, Vishwanath Sardesai, CRC Press, p. 19.

Chapter 1

Scotland and Ireland

January

Weight 1-3-11: 256.5 lbs. Hgb A1C 8.8

Weight 1-8-11: 249 lbs.

Weight 2-2-11: 258 lbs. after trip to Ireland and Scotland. Mostly, a car tour with little exercise.

Baseline lab before very low-carb diet

LDL-P 651

LDL-C 70

Tubby Factor 82

Insulin resistance 45

ApoB 62

Small LDL-P < 90

LDL size 21.3

HDL-C 51

HDL-P 33.9

Triglycerides 62

Lab done 8-28-10 while on Crestor 5 mg, Endur-acin 1,000 mg, and Lovaza 4,000 mg.

I was at Sheraton Mountain Vista Timeshare in Avon, Colorado, during the first week of January. There were record low temperatures when I had an epiphany: carbohydrates drive insulin, which drives hunger and fat accumulation. The source of the revelation was Gary Taubes's book, *Why We Get Fat: And What to Do About It*.

I decided to make myself a case study of one. I would go on a very low-carbohydrate diet for a year and follow my advanced lipid panel several times over the course of the year with a repeat CIMT and CAC at the end of the year.

Guinness in Ireland and Scotland

During the second week of January, I lost 7 lbs. as I started the very low-carb diet of 20 g of carbohydrate a day.

On January 12, we flew to Philadelphia and stayed with friends for three nights. I found I could stay on my low-carb diet easily. I missed the Philly cheesesteaks of Dalesandro's, but I made up for it with chicken wings and Manhattan cocktails at the local bars. No formal exercise, but we usually walked like tourists every day.

A real challenge to the dieter is a transatlantic flight. So much so that usually people give up on their diets for that very boring period of forced inactivity. I was in the early phase of my diet and still very motivated. I didn't eat the carbs but drank wine to help pass the time. The forced sedentary life is extremely bad for diets. It does something to the metabolism. I will get into that later.

We arrived in Glasgow Airport on January 15, rented a car, and drove to the Scottish Highlands. More forced sedentary life in a car. Very bad. Who goes to Scotland in January? Scotland just had the worse December weather in 100 years. Days are short. The sun doesn't get very high in the sky. Look at a map. It is much farther north than my birthplace in NYC. It is warmer than NYC because of the Gulf Stream. Travel has taught me much. While we were in Scotland and Ireland, it never went below freezing. The struggle was the lack of sunlight. It was like Seattle with the drizzling rain. We had some sun one day. We loved it. No tourist crowds. A true traveler takes it as it comes and doesn't whine. This weather was made for poets. "A Man Is a Man for All That," Robert Burns. I would sing "My Love Is Like a Red Red Rose" to my wife. After the third time, she said, "Enough." We did mostly driving and less walking on this part of our trip. The landscape is similar to Vermont but with less trees and more heather. The Scottish Highlands is one of the most beautiful places in the world. We stayed in Aviemore at a Hilton timeshare. We knew we would get an electric bill at the end of the week. We kept our cabin temperature very low. They still charged us $70 for the electricity. We went to the top of Craggenmore Mountain for the second time in our lives. Last time was in June and it was cold and raining. This time we were very lucky. It was cold but sunny! The Scots were skiing on the snow slopes. Wow! What a special day. Some locals told us they wanted Scotland to be independent of England. They were not happy with the British royalty. The Avis car rental ripped us off by charging us 100 lbs. for a bump in the tire. Oh, Mr. Burns, what has happened to Scotland? First, the electricity overcharge and then the rental car scam.

Eating in Scotland on a low-carb diet was not difficult except for the Guinness. I was required to drink Guinness by tradition. I am not a beer drinker, but it may be impossible to get a Manhattan cocktail in a pub. I think the lack of exercise and sitting in the car with the carbs from stout beer prevented me from losing weight. The Scottish breakfast is good for the protein, but I passed up the blood sausage. I will eat haggis but not the blood sausage.

We flew to Dublin, Ireland, on January 22. The Guinness brewery was a great tourist trap, and there was free beer at the top of Dublin. Unforgettable. It is very important to learn a proper pour of Guinness. I also researched how many carbs in Guinness stout—16 g. Not good for my low-carb diet. However, when you visit the oldest pub in Ireland at Athelone and meet the famous Irish artist Paul Proud, there is no choice but to share a Guinness with him.

When I returned to Kansas on February 2, I weighed 258 lbs. again. At fifteen years old, I went on the Weight Watchers diet. It worked well for me. I dieted over the years on different diets. In 2005, I went on insulin. I was 250 lbs. A year later, I was 280 lbs. In March 2006, I went on the *Three-Hour Diet* by Jorge Cruise. This was a great diet for me because I could eat a 300-calorie snack between meals. The three-hour diet is a hypocalorie diet. I lost 80 lbs. by 6-30-07, the day of my wedding.

My metabolism had hit rock bottom. I could not lose any more weight despite two hours of exercise a day. I decided to gain some weight back to build up some muscle so I could increase my metabolism.

I read *The Skinny On Losing Weight Without Being Hungry* by Louis J. Aronne. I followed his advice and started eating the equivalent of four egg whites for breakfast each morning. I exercised up to three hours a day. I was retired. I did forty-five minutes of water aerobics three times a week. I walked on the treadmill every day or took an hour walk. I did weight lifting every day, alternating legs with upper body. I hired two trainers and worked out with them a few times a week.

I continued to gain weight until January 2011. I read *Why We Get Fat: And What to Do about It* by Gary Taubes. I decided to go on 20 g of carbohydrates a day. I also tried to eat 30 g of protein with each meal. This meant I would eat 60% fat a day.

This book is about eating low-carb diet while taking six cruises over ninety days.

I continued to drink alcohol.

I decreased my exercise to less than an hour a day.

This is a unique case study about a bon vivant (myself) who traveled 200 days on the road and on the sea eating and drinking extremely well.

Science Section

I respect Dr. Louis J. Aronne and think he wrote a very good book entitled *The Skinny On Losing Weight Without Being Hungry*. On page 23 he writes, "If you consume too much rapidly digested carbohydrate at once, insulin levels rise too high and drive down blood sugar levels too quickly, leading to rebound hunger and interfering with the leptin-signaling mechanism, leading to leptin resistance. Another gut hormone called glucose-dependent insulinotropic peptide (GIP) also rises when you consume starch, and it rises faster and more dramatically when you consume rapidly digested starch. This gut hormone is responsible for gauging when starch comes in too quickly for body cells to burn. High levels of GIP flip a fat-storage switch. They start the conversion of starch into triglycerides (fat) and signal fat cells to soak up this fat from the bloodstream."

"One way to reverse fullness resistance, reduce hunger and discourage fat storage is to consume carbohydrate foods that result in slow and gradual rises in both insulin and GIP."

This is what I tried, but I think grapes, cherries, apples, plums, pears, and bananas were a source of carbs that caused me to gain 1.5 lbs. a month despite two hours of exercise a day. See the chapter on Fat Wars. I ate these "healthy" foods because I thought my exercise would burn off the extra calories. It didn't. I don't think differentiating between low-or high-glycemic carbs makes a difference. See the Brazilian bean study cited in the chapter on Fat Wars.

Carbohydrates drive insulin, which drives fat accumulation and hunger. The way to avoid this is to eat only 20 g of carbohydrates a day.

I do believe fat people have more cancer. Thus, if a fat person loses weight with a high-fat diet, he will have less chances of getting cancer. Weight loss is more important than eating antioxidants. The evidence of the effectiveness of antioxidants is theoretical while that of weight loss is much stronger. Eating saturated fat does not cause cancer. Being fat puts you at increased risk of cancer. I will discuss recent articles that suggest processed meat does pose a health risk.

Lipid instruction

For nonmedical readers, I suggest you focus only on the LDL-P number in this book. My goal is to get my LDL-P to 750 or lower. The AIM trial has shown that HDL-C and triglycerides are not of primary importance once the LDL-C is at goal.

This is what I was taught by Dr. Dayspring and what I wrote in my book *The Tubby Theory from Topeka*. Once the LDL-P is at 750, it is not important to try to get the HDL-C or the triglycerides to certain goals. However, for lipid geeks, the fun is in the details of the advanced lipid test. Physicians have very little knowledge of the liposcience report or the VAP report.

I hope my case study will help physicians and the general public to learn how to interpret these advanced lipid tests. LDL-C is the old standard. It is the amount of cholesterol in the blood. LDL-P and apoB measure the number of atherogenic particles. This is the best predictor of disease.

The Tubby Factor is the term I coined for non-HDL cholesterol. It is a better predictor than the LDL-C number but not better than the particle number. The good thing about the Tubby Factor is that there is no extra cost for this. Look at your old lipid panel. Subtract the HDL from the total cholesterol. It should be less than eighty if you want plaque regression.

CRPhs and PLAC2 are blood tests to measure inflammation. I will not talk much about CRPhs and PLAC2 because it is my experience that once you get the LDL-P down to 750, the inflammation parameters are usually good. There is no specific treatment for the high CRPhs other than statins. Once the LDL-P is at 750, you would not want to increase the statin. You may want to maximize the fish oil to Lovaza 4,000 mg a day. I think everyone should take DHA and EPA of 850 mg a day.

This case study has five end points:

1. Weight
2. LDL-P
3. CIMT
4. CAC
5. Hemoglobin A1C

I previously showed regression in my CAC and CIMT in my book *The Tubby Theory from Topeka*. Let's see what happens to my diabetes and plaque after twelve months of 60% fat.

Tubby Thought

Sedentary Danger

"Men who reported more than 23 hours a week of sedentary activity(other than sleeping 8 hours a day) had a 64% greater risk of dying from heart disease than those who reported less than 11 hours a week of sedentary activity. Many of these men routinely exercised. They recommended hourly mini-breaks, even 1 minute long throughout the day helps movement of muscles and provide health benefits" (Vishwanath Sardesai, *Introduction to Clinical Nutrition,* 3rd edition [CRC Press], pp. 19-20).

Chapter 2

Florida

February

Weight 2-1-11: 258 lbs.
Weight 2-10-11: 256 lbs.

We left cold Kansas for sunny Florida on February 11. It took three days and two nights to get to our timeshare in Bonnet Creek, Disney World. This sedentary activity of driving all day is extremely bad. The discipline to exercise after the mental fatigue of driving ten hours is as difficult as staying on a low-calorie diet for more than five years.

The timeshare has a kitchen. Low-carb diet is easy when you control what you buy at the grocery store. I had been to the theme parks many times. You definitely do not want to eat at them no matter what diet you are on. I love the parks. I would take my kids to the gates of the theme parks before they opened. Once we were let in, we would race through the rides before there were long lines. We would go home for lunch at noon as the lines became impossible.

We went to Universal to see the Harry Potter exhibit. The area for Harry Potter is closed off once it gets too crowded. We were there early enough to not wait to get into the area. It is very nice, and the premiere ride is excellent. I thought it was a little better than the Spiderman ride, which had been rated the best adventure ride in Orlando.

We then went to another timeshare at Jensen Beach for thirteen days. Again, I had no difficulty following my low-carb diet at the timeshare. I had a kitchen and ate three eggs with three strips of bacon every morning. We purchased cold cuts with mayonnaise and pickles for lunch and the cooked steak or chicken or hamburger or hot dogs for dinner with a large salad and blue cheese dressing. I was never hungry, and I could be satisfied with three meals a day. We watched a beautiful sunset each night with a homemade Manhattan. We walked a little on the beach most days.

We left for New Orleans on March 3. More driving, ugh. As the title page quote states, I needed "hourly mini-breaks, even 1 minute long throughout the day to help movement of muscles and provide health benefits."

Science Section

People who run marathons are not immune from heart disease. Jim Fixx is a good example of a marathon runner who suffered from sudden cardiac death. Arthur Ash was also thin and a professional tennis player who had severe heart disease. Often at marathons, there are deaths from cardiovascular disease.

Fact one: Everyone can lose weight. Only 5% can maintain the weight after five years.

Fact two: Only marathon runners can prevent weight gain as they get older; otherwise, exercise does not maintain long-term weight loss.

Fact three: Behavior, willpower, and counting calories do not cure obesity.

Fact four: No one knows what has caused the obesity epidemic.

Fact five: No one can prove that they know what a healthy diet is.

Fact six: A healthy diet may have nothing to do with what you eat but how you cook it. How you cook your food determines how much advanced glycolation end products (AGE) are in it. These are proinflammatory substances.

Tubby Thought

Willpower

"Putting individual solutions and free will up against the increase in portion sizes, massive technological and societal changes, food-company taste-engineering, and the ubiquity of effective television advertisements is like asking Ecuador to conquer China. And yet that is what public-health campaigns suggest we do" (Marc Ambinder, "Fat Nation: It's Worse Than You Think. How to Beat Obesity," *The Atlantic* [May 2010], pp. 78-79).

Chapter 3

Mardi Gras and Texas

March

Weight 2-10-11: 256 lbs.
Weight 3-14-11: 254 lbs. after a thirty-one-day road trip and minimal exercise
Weight 3-18-11: 255.5 lbs.

LDL-P 1,246 (goal < 750)
LDL-C 110 (goal < 70)
Tubby Factor 127 (goal < 80)
Insulin resistance 37 (goal? < 27)
ApoB 81 (goal < 60)
Small LDL-P 408 (goal? < 117)
LDL size 21.5 nm (goal > 20.8)
HDL-C 58 (goal > 40)
HDL-P 37.2 (goal > 35)
Triglycerides 83 (goal < 100)
(Lab done on 3-12-11 in Austin, Texas.)

We arrived in New Orleans just in time for Mardi Gras on March 6. We stayed at the W for five days on Starwood points as the fifth night was free. My son was living in New Orleans, and we partied hard with him and his friends. Most people don't realize that the parades don't go through Bourbon Street. Mardi Gras is actually a family event although most people are drinking alcohol. We found kids throwing footballs in the streets between parades, and there were many ladders with seats on the top for the little kids to see the parade better. The people on the floats gave out special treats to kids.

Our favorite eating place was LUKE. They have an oyster happy hour. Perfect for the brave low-carb dieter. I say brave because you can't tell a bad oyster by looking at it. Vibrio can contaminate the raw oysters and make you sick. If you are immune compromised, it can kill you. Hey, this is the Big Easy. I ate thirty-six oysters in one sitting with two Manhattans and one classic gin martini with olives. We went there at least three times during the five days. The low-carb diet is restrictive, and I avoided the po'boy sandwiches, but I was not hungry, so I did not feel deprived.

I highly recommend going to the WWII museum. After that, go through district nine to see the work that has been done to repair the damage from Hurricane Katrina. If you like music, watch the TV box set called Treme. It is about the recovery in New Orleans. Excellent music and an excellent show.

On March 11 we drove to Austin to attend the National Lipid Association meeting. I heard Dr. Superko present his study of Atlanta firefighters. He screened them with CAC and found many fireman with low Framingham scores (low-cardiac event risk) to have significant plaque. That is the tubby project that I tried to initiate in Topeka but failed to get any interest in it. I was happy to see that someone accomplished it with good results.

At the NLA meeting, I had advanced lipid testing done. I was very disappointed with the results. My LDL-P went up. I think the Guinness and all the driving and flying contributed to this. I had not lost significant weight. I did not give up because my main goal was to lower my Hgb A1C. This did happen. I decided I would exercise more on the cruise and would increase my Crestor if I needed to.

We drove home to Topeka on March 13. We had to get ready to fly to Hong Kong.

Lab Section

I started a very low-carb diet after reading Gary Taubes's book, *Why We Get Fat*, around January 5, 2011. I decreased my metformin from 2,000 mg to 1,000 mg. My Hgb A1C dropped from 8.7 to 8.2 and then 7.9. On 5-16-11, my Hgb A1C was 7.7 after forty-five days on cruise.

In Austin, I had a VAP and Liposcience done around March 7, 2011. These are advanced lipid blood testing by two different companies.

VAP non-HDL chol = 119

Liposcience non-HDL cholesterol = 185—58 = 123

The best Tubby Factor score is less than eighty to regress plaque in arteries.

More March data

My LDL-P went from 600 to 1,248. This was very disturbing to see after six weeks of low-carb diet. I think the long hours of driving had much to do with it. There was little exercise during this road trip.

My apoB (VAP) went from 60 to 85. This is a fairly good apoB result. My liposcience LDL-P of 1,268 might be considered highly discordant with the calculated apoB of the VAP.

It may be that an apoB is not as accurate as the LDL-P in people with metabolic syndrome.

Lipid instruction

My opinion is that my LDL-P went up because I gained 6 pounds. and not because I was on a low-carbohydrate diet. I did not lose heart because my Hgb A1C went down despite decreasing my metformin from 2,000 mg to 1,000 mg. If my next LDL-P was elevated, my plan was to increase my Crestor from 5 mg to 10 mg. My insulin resistance number was 37. This was lower than my IR 45 in August 2010 when I was not on a low-carb diet.

I had 60% fat in my diet and most of that fat was animal fat. The "low-fat diet" people (Ornish) would say that their LDL-C goes down when they lose weight. There is the confounding covariable argument. Not only is total fat reduced in their weight loss diets, carbohydrates are also reduced. Often in low-fat diets the HDL-C goes down and the triglycerides go up.

The Atkins folks (low-carb diet) would say that while the LDL-C goes up in their diets, the LDL particles are larger and fluffier, putting the patient in pattern A. This, they claim, is less atherogenic than the small, dense particles that the low-fat diet produces.

Indeed, on my low-carb diet, my HDL-C did go up from 51 in August 2010 to 58. However, I contend that the LDL-P number is what matters the most. What is very interesting is that not only did the HDL-C go up but my HDL-P number went up by 3.3 points. This type of data is just not available in the present lipid trials to my knowledge, and yet it is crucial information.

The LDL size did not change much for me on the two diets. I suspect it is because I am on four Lovaza a day. This is the correction the low-fat diets are trying to make to change their pattern from B (small LDL) to A (large fluffy LDL). Again, the latest evidence is that size is not that important. The number of particles is most important.

My small LDL particle number shot up from less than 90 in August to 408 on a low-carb diet. Again, I believe the particle number went up because I was sedentary for long periods driving the car. Driving for ten hours, stopping for gas only three times is very bad for the muscles. (See quote on Tubby Thought p. 38.)

I will follow all these variables in the coming year, and by the end of the book, I hope the reader will know the lipid jargon.

Tubby Thought

Resistance Training Is Good but Not Essential

Tim Church's Ultimate Workout:
High intensity one day a week
Resistance training (weights) one to two days a week
Aerobic forty-five to sixty minutes a day
Stretching four to five days a week
Presented at the Core Conference at the obesity meeting in Orlando in October 2011.

Caveat emptor:

"Weight lifting has virtually no effect on resting metabolism . . . If the man lifts weights and gains 2.2 kg (4.4 lbs.) of muscle, his metabolic rate would increase by 24 calories a day" (Claude Bouchard as related by Gina Kolata in her book, *Ultimate Fitness* [2003], p. 230).

Chapter 4

Hong Kong to Athens Cruise

April

Weight: none done at official scale at home while on cruise for the whole month

We stepped up to first-class flight. We used our Starwood points to do it in an affordable manner. We purchased Westin Lagunar Mar timeshare. We pay a yearly maintenance fee of $1,400. If we convert the two-bedroom locked-off room to Starwood points, we get 80,000 points each year. We get a bonus of 20,000 points because of our platinum status. We then deposit our Starwood points into frequent-flier miles. We can get a first-class ticket for 100,000 frequent-flier points with British Airlines, Virgin Airlines, American Airlines, and Iberia Airlines. The other airlines may charge up to 150,000 frequent-flier miles for first class. Business class will be less. We used our Starwood points to fly first-class to Hong Kong. It was wonderful. We stretched out on a chair that opened to a flat surface. I never slept so well on a plane. The airfare without points can range from $3,000 to $13,000. After ten to twenty flights, we figure we will break even on the initial outlay for the Mexican timeshare. Most important, the points are supposedly inflation resistant except for the maintenance fee going up. If you understood all this, you will have no trouble with the science sections.

For forty-five days, we were on Oceana Cruise from Hong Kong to Athens. There are two specialty restaurants on the *Nautica*. One is a steak grill that made a 32 oz. rib roast–perfect for a low-carb diet. The other restaurant is Italian. Yes, it was difficult to forgo all the wonderful pasta. However, the osso buco and veal milanese more than made up for it. The waiter would bring a cart with numerous types of olive oil and vinegars. I admit I did have this with a little of their wonderful bread but not often and not much.

Chinese food is a big disappointment. A low-carb dieter can get by with Peking duck at the Spring Restaurant in Hong Kong. Other than that, there is McDonald's. Eat the double cheeseburgers without the buns. Shanghai is a place where everyone must eat the dumplings or dim sum. It has the best dim sum in the world. I had eaten it during a prior trip.

Vietnam has better food than China and more protein friendly, especially fish and shrimp.

Vietnam has the fastest growing economy in the world. They want to be the next China. They have no grudges about the American War (as they call it); after all, they won it. Their war museum shows what we did to their people with Agent Orange. It upsets some of the Americans. Other than that, it is all bygones with the Vietnamese people. Watch out for those motorcycles. Fifty deaths a day in Saigon (no one calls it Ho Chi Min City). We purchased a beautiful cherry tree lacquer panel from a factory here. We mailed it home. Good value for a beautiful piece. A friend purchased large jewels here at a good price.

Singapore was a disappointment. Perhaps we were not there long enough. I had such high expectations. The architecture was mostly sterile apartment buildings. People who had been there twenty years ago said it was much more exotic and better back then.

Phuket, Thailand, was a natural wonderland.

Myanmar switched to a civilian government while we were there. We asked the locals what it meant. They had no idea. There was no Internet while we were there as with the Chinese; it was all shut down because of the Arab Spring.

We spent two nights and three days in Burma. From the ship, we could see seven Buddhist temples in the distance. The ship was docked in a very rural area. We saw quite a few giant Buddhas. A great deal of money was spent on these statues. We purchased a beautiful tapestry here. We packed it and carried it home. Our friend purchased a large ruby and other large gemstones at a low price. Food was similar to Vietnam but not quite as good.

Next stop was India. Cochin was a surprise. An ancient port with Chinese nets still used for fishing. There was a Christian church founded by St. Thomas that was there when Gambo explored the area for Portugal. We did not eat in Cochin or Mumbai. India was not the mess I thought it was going to be. There were stray cows walking around. Cochin was very tolerant of the Christian and Jewish population. Muslims and Hindus lived with them peacefully. I will go back to India. There are twenty-two provinces and they are all very different.

We then prepared to go through the pirate seas. The *Nautica* had fended off a prior attack and made world news. Our captain gave an interesting talk on pirates. Despite our fears, there was no pirate attack. In truth, the pirates do not seem very formidable. We had five Israelis on board hired to protect us from an attack. They were part of a security company. The captain had once chased off the pirates with an ear-splitting sonic weapon. We also had fire hose on the decks to fire at the aluminum ladders the pirates would use. No guns on board apparently.

Next stop, the Middle East. I learned a lot here and on our visit to Israel but that is for a different book. In our travels we saw few fat people. Asians seem to have a genetic protection from obesity. No nation seemed to be starving. Indians develop metabolic syndrome when they move to America. I think it is from our high intake of carbs. Middle East folks are getting fatter, but we didn't see them. The high-carb diets are causing a great deal of diabetes in Saudi Arabia. In the rich Arab nations, the Arabs prefer to hire Indians and Pakistanis to do the physical labor.

I love the days at sea. It is also a good opportunity to exercise. I usually walk at least eight minutes on the deck after each meal. Often, I do at least twenty minutes and sometimes as much as sixty minutes on the deck. Walking with the ocean all around is wonderful. We don't get that in Kansas. My wife and I always take the steps on the ship. I have determined this is our intense interval training and may boost our metabolism. I usually do not gain weight after cruises.

Tubby Thought

Obesity is 40-70% genetics. Mickey Stunkard discovered this many years ago with twin studies.

Caveat emptor:

"Why do we still blame the fat for being fat?" (Moral Hazard)

Chapter 5

Barhopping in New York City

May

    Weight 3-18-11: 255.5 lbs.
    Weight 5-17-11: 257 lbs. after forty-five days in the Oceania cruise
    Weight 5-27-11: 254 lbs.

    LDL-P 765 (goal < 750)
    LDL-C 55 (goal < 70)
    Tubby Factor 64 (goal < 80)
    Insulin resistance 25 (goal? < 27)
    ApoB 67 (goal < 60)
    Small LDL-P 363 (goal? < 117)
    LDL size 21.5 nm (goal? > 20.8)
    HDL-C 61 (goal > 40)
    HDL-P 35.7 (goal > 35)
    Triglycerides 45 (goal < 100)

    (Lab done on 5-20-11 in NYC after a forty-five-day cruise.)

We returned from Athens to Topeka on May 12. We flew to Spain and changed planes to fly to Chicago. Again, the first-class leg across the ocean was wonderful.

However, the whole trip took twenty-four hours to get door-to-door. Even first class couldn't prevent the fatigue from that effort.

I was delighted that I ate all I wanted and yet did not gain significant weight after forty-five days on a cruise ship. A low-carbohydrate diet is easy to follow on a cruise ship. The first twenty-two days I actually lost 8 lbs. because I did not drink. The second half of the trip, we started drinking wine and made cocktails in our room as we watched the sunsets from our veranda. I suspect alcohol is the main reason I have not lost much weight on the low-carb diet. Hey, I was retired and on vacation. I partied and I didn't get hungry and I didn't gain weight. More importantly, my Hgb A1C continued to go lower and my lipid panel went back to its excellent level. On May 18, I flew to NYC to attend another National Lipid Association meeting. I had my advanced lipid studies done and they were quite good. I took my twenty-seven-year-old son with me, and we went barhopping. I like to visit the old bars, but this time we enjoyed the Bull and Bear in the Waldorf Astoria. Very elegant. The cigar bar across the bar from Carnegie Hall was very cozy. The most fun was to find the Campbell Apartment bar in Grand Central Station. The Flatiron bar was more modern and for a younger crowd. It was my least favorite. NYC is all about the food. I missed not eating knishes and pizza. We had a kebab on Eight Avenue in an Afghan restaurant. Very reasonable price.

The NLA has a Web site—Lipid.org. Some nutritionists had complained that the August meeting in Washington did not serve "healthy food." Subsequently, the next meeting had no eggs and bacon for breakfast. As a diabetic, the granola was the worst thing I could eat. I had to eat hard-boiled eggs. Nutrition Nazis who don't know what they are talking about. A low-fat diet is not necessarily a healthy diet for Tubbies, the diabetic, or people with metabolic syndrome. There is no evidence that antioxidants A, C, or E do any magic for our health in high dose. It is just theory that has failed to be proven in several trials. In Arbiter, vitamin E showed a bad outcome on statins. Of course, the critics said it was the wrong type of vitamin E. Food religion is very fervent.

How can you eat a lot of fat and not have your cholesterol (LDL-C) go up?

In the absolutely correct mathematical skinny world, it just doesn't make sense that a high-fat diet doesn't cause high cholesterol or more heart attacks. More amazing is the fact that in the tubby world, a low-carb diet helps people with the tubby syndrome (metabolic syndrome) or diabetes more than a low-fat diet because in the tubby world the golden rule is carbs drive insulin, which drives fat accumulation.

In my last book, *The Tubby Theory from Topeka*, I presented the tubby diet. I initially admitted that diet was a stumbling block or deal breaker. However, I thought the tubby diet was an exact way that involved little preparation as it included frozen foods that could be microwaved. I meticulously listed the percentage of saturated fat with the usual guidelines, advising 35% fat and 7% saturated fat and almost no trans fat. I thought that the portion control of preprepared food and the ease of preparation might help some people with a low-calorie diet.

After five years, I have continued to be 10% less than my original weight. However, I gained back 50 lbs. despite two hours of exercise a day. My LDL-P was not going up with weight gain, but my Hgb A1C was going up. I went from 6.5 to 8.7. In January 2011, I read Gary Taubes's book, *Why We Get Fat*. It was an epiphany for me. I immediately started a low-carb diet. After two months, my LDL-P went from 600 to 1,200. I was quite concerned. I was driving around the country, and my exercise routine was about nil. However, my Hgb A1C went down with half of the usual metformin. I was delighted, and I had not gained weight, and I was not hungry. This was what I was looking for. I could always take more statins if my LDL-P stayed above 1,000.

The next two months I spent circumnavigating the world. I caught an Oceania cruise ship in Hong Kong and was taken to Athens. I exercised quite a bit. During days at sea, I walked the deck two to three times a day, eight to sixty minutes each time. I also always took the steps, not the elevator, and did some weight lifting. I did some walking on the tours when in port. At 250-plus pounds, walking three to five flights is intense interval training.

I ate very well. I had eggs and bacon each morning. I ate osso buco and a 32 oz. bone in prime rib three times. I had fish once.

I didn't gain significant weight once I checked myself at home on my usual scale.

Tubby Thought

Resting Metabolic Rate

"Basal Metabolic rate accounts for ~70% of daily energy expenditure, whereas active physical activity contributes 5%-10%. Thus, a significant component of daily energy consumption is fixed" (Longo et al., *Harrison's Principles of Internal Medicine*, 18th edition [McGraw Hill], p. 623).

Chapter 6

Hawaii

June

Weight 5-27-11: 254 lbs.
Weight 6-27-11: 252.5 lbs. after twenty-nine days in Hawaii

We flew first-class to Hawaii on Delta on 5-29-11. It was a terrible experience. They changed our itineraries so that we had to travel about twenty-four hours to get to Hawaii. The first-class portion from Milwaukee to Honolulu was good, but we arrived late and had to get a later flight to Maui. The most egregious deeds by Delta were committed when we returned to Kansas. They cancelled our first-class status. We had made the reservations a year ago and Delta confirmed our status the day before we left. Unbelievable that other people were given our first-class seats. When I complained, the supervisor called security to stand by. We made twenty phone calls, and they finally refunded some of our points. They were going to keep all the extra frequent-flier points we had used to upgrade to first class without a refund to us.

We stayed at timeshares again. We stayed at a deluxe oceanfront one-bedroom apartment at Diamond Resort on North Ka'anapali. With a kitchen, a low-carb diet is not difficult. Maui is the best as it has a sunset view of the ocean with Lanai and Molokai in the distance. January to March is the time to go to see the 2,000 humpback whales right from your window. Whales and rainbows. What could be better? Oh, yes, waterfalls when you drive to Hana. We drove to Hana and spent two nights there. We left Hana and took the unpaved road around the mountain. Rental car companies do not want you to do this, but I did not find it very difficult. Finally, there is the volcano. I hiked into the bottom of the crater and climbed out. Very arduous for this old man. Going down was easy but climbing out of the crater in never-ending switchback trails and being low on water exhausted me. The whole hike took eight hours. It was worth it. I did it with my youngest son, who found it to be a breeze. He saved my life by giving me some of his water. When we got back to the car, I was dehydrated and drank a cup of leftover coffee. It was ambrosia in my condition. I let my son drive down the mountain. Another infraction with the rental company. Breaking the rules when traveling is sometimes unavoidable.

The road to Hana has a smoothie place with fresh fruit. Hawaii is all about fruit. Fruit is anathema for low-carb dieters. I just sucked it up and did not yield to temptation. Fruit is called healthy. The fruit of modern man is genetically chosen to be very high in glucose. It is not healthy for a diabetic. Orange juice is liquid sugar. It is not healthy food.

We flew to Kauai for the last two weeks of our trip. We stayed at the St. Regis Hotel at Princeville with our Starwood points. We got a free upgrade as part of our platinum status, and it turned out to be the nicest place we have ever stayed at. We had a junior suite with a view of the Hanalei Bay that was outstanding. The waterfalls would spring up after each rain cloud passed.

I found my food source to be Bubba's when we did not have a kitchen. The triple burger was great. I did not eat the bun. There are three Bubba's on Kauai, and I ate at each one. The final two weeks, we stayed at a timeshare at Poipu. The good news is the Hawaiian green turtles are back. They are thinking of taking them off the extinction list. Every day we saw several off shore.

Tubby Thought

Hey, Joe, Say It Ain't So

p. 1202:
"Little Progress has been made in prevention or treatment (of obesity) . . ."
p. 1204:
"Using conventional dietary techniques only 20% of patients will lose 20 lb.
and maintain the loss for over 2 years; 5% will maintain a 40 lb loss."

Robert B. Baron, MD, MS
2011 *Current Medical Diagnosis and Treatment*
Stephen J. McPhee, McGraw Hill, LANGE

Chapter 7

European River Cruise

July

Weight 6-27-11: 252.5 lbs.
Weight 7-26-11: 253 lbs. after the European river cruise

We left for Amsterdam on June 29. We stayed at the Pulitzer for two nights before we boarded the *Viking Prestige* riverboat. Our itinerary was to sail all the way to Bucharest, Romania, in twenty-one days. We were looking forward to eating the different foods and wines of the several countries we were passing through. Once on board, they offered us the Silver Beverage Plan. For $300, we had unlimited wine and alcohol from a full bar for fourteen days. We met two other couples who were on the same plan, and we partied every day. It was the most fun I ever had on a ship. The wine was great. For someone who only started drinking seriously two years ago, I was amazed I never got sick. We certainly drank our $300 without difficulty. The remaining seven days of our cruise, we switched to the *Prima Dona* and did not join the plan. After all that drinking, I did not gain weight. The river cruise was very different from the ocean cruise. The ship was much smaller with only 150 passengers. The river cruise was good except that there were no exercise facilities. I did very little exercise during those twenty-one days. The top deck had an area to walk around on, but most of the time the passengers were forbidden to go up there because the deck was broken down to allow the boat to pass under low bridges. We had no days at sea, and we did have a tour every day. It was usually a half-day tour and not very strenuous.

The low-carbohydrate diet was easy to follow on this cruise. The salad bar was superb. There were 1,000 different sausages from Germany. Sirloin steak was offered as an alternative to the new nightly menu. I took advantage of the sirloin three times. The meals were not large portions at night, but they often came around and offered extra fish or meat if there was some leftover. Overall, the food on the riverboat never reached the zeniths that the specialty restaurants achieved on the ocean liner, but the food was good and fresh. The entertainment and talks were minimal, but they tried. The crew was very friendly on both riverboats.

The river cruise had windmills, castles, cathedrals, and medieval towns, but the best part was two stretches on the Rhine where we would spend the afternoon in the sun on the top deck, enjoying the scenery of the mountains on either side as the waiters served us drinks. This was one of my best travel experiences.

Tubby Thought

The Government Knows How to Prevent Obesity?

"Our public health leaders must replace prevarication with imagination" (from the editorial concerning obesity–"The Catastrophic Failures of Public Health," Lancet [2004], pp. 363-745).

Caveat emptor:

"Two large studies in the 1990s, for example, asked whether the measures usually advocated to prevent children from gaining weight are effective."

See:
Benjamin Caballero did an eight-year, $20-million project sponsored by National Heart, Lung, and Blood Institute with 1,704 third graders in the Southwest (*American Journal of Clinical Nutrition* [2003]).

Also:
Archives of Pediatrics and Adolescent Medicine in 1999.
Around 5,106 children from ninety-six schools in California, Louisiana, Michigan, and Texas sponsored by the National Institutes of Health.

In neither of these large studies did government intervention help prevent obesity (Gina Kolata, *Rethinking Thin*, pp. 197-199).

Chapter 8

Paradise Island, Atlantis, Bahamas

August

> Weight 8-4-11: 251.5 lbs.
> Weight 8-7-11: 249 lbs., a new low for the year of 2011

On August 7, we drove two of our cars loaded with stuff like the Beverly Hillbillies to our new residence in Jensen Beach, Florida. We had our dog, Cosmo, with us. It took two nights and three days, but all went well except for the total sedentary lifestyle driving like that imposes.

What excitement to set up a new home in a condo overlooking the ocean. We were busy buying furniture and getting our Florida driver's licenses. No time to use the condo gym or golf course. On August 13, we flew to Nassau from Fort Lauderdale on Spirit. This flight was $200 cheaper than flying out of West Palm Springs, but Spirit charges $42 for the first bag and $50 for a second bag. This is the flight the Bahamians take to bring all their USA purchases back to the island. Apparently, it is much cheaper than buying these items on their island, or the items are not even available. As in Hawaii, island living is very expensive.

We stayed at our timeshare at Harborside, Atlantis. We took a taxi for $40 to the grocery store to buy food to cook for the week. We purchased a turkey and cooked it in our kitchen. Roasting a big turkey in the oven at a timeshare makes the place smell like home. I love the roasted skin, and there is plenty of protein for the rest of the week. The groceries are expensive. Still cooking in the timeshare is much cheaper than eating out three times a day. We ate out one night at the Dune restaurant. For four people without drinks the bill was $260. The food was excellent.

We returned to our new home in Florida and sought out a new physician in Jensen Beach in order to be plugged into the health system while we stayed there during the winter months. I asked him to do a glucose finger stick. To my shock and dismay, I had a postprandial glucose of 340. Then my Hgb A1C came back at 10.3. My low-carbohydrate diet had failed me. In May, I had gone off Actos on the advice of a "low-carb diet" specialist. Over the next three months, I noticed that my abdomen became firmer. I believe the fat moved from the periphery to central fat. Actos also was shown to contribute to some congestive heart failure because of peripheral edema. Since I haven't had heart failure, I didn't think that was a concern for me. I immediately increased my metformin to 2,000 mg a day and went back on Actos 45 mg. That was on July 24. On July 26, I attended a National Lipid Association meeting in Orlando. I would get my lipid panel and discover if my lipids had gone awry as well.

The Battle of Orlando

I was at the National Lipid Association meeting. After hearing a speaker say, "We all know high-fat diets are associated with more coronary diseases," I had to speak up.

At the question segment, I said I had four things to say:

1. First, I wanted to apologize for what I was going to say.
2. I was very disappointed in the talk. We have an obesity epidemic, and I was being told to eat healthy exotic snacks instead of junk food. I haven't had junk food since 2006.
3. I have been on a 60% fat diet, mostly animal fat, and my lipid profile was excellent.
4. I have been on a low-carb diet since January, and my Hgb A1C improved as a result, and I had decreased my exercise.

An eminent professor got up and said that he remembered seeing people on the Atkins diet with cholesterols of 300. I replied that was anecdotal. The A-Z trial by Gardner and the comparative diet trial by Sachs both showed that Atkins was lipid neutral. We had a Afro-American professor that spoke earlier who agreed with me that carbs were a problem with blacks and Hispanics. We had an Asian

Indian professor who said that Indians ate a contaminated vegetarian diet and that much of that was probably carbs that pushed them into the metabolic syndrome.

Concerning the Prevarication Quote

Large public health studies have been done and appear to be ignored by public health officials.

NIH study: 5,100 kids in third grade reported in 1999, p. 199, in *Rethinking Thin* by Gina Kolata

"The largest school-based random based trial ever conducted." The Archives of Pediatrics and Adolescent Medicine in 1999.

Result: The children ate less fat and exercised more. These children's weights were no different from those of children in schools that served as controls.

NIH study by Benjamin Caballero was published in *American Journal of Clinical Nutrition* in 2003.

The children decreased the fat intake in their diet from 34% to 27%. However, after two years, it was not enough to change the body weight in 1,704 third graders. These two large, intense intervention trials seem to be forgotten, as written by Gina Kolata.

"Our public health leaders must replace prevarication with imagination" (Lancet editorial, March 6, 2004, volume 363, number 9411, p. 745).

Michelle Obama has a Let's Move initiative. In her White House kitchen staff, the pastry chef is now riding her bike 13 miles a day and is losing weight. I hope she learns about the reduced obese state and the subsequent development of the Sponge Syndrome.

Tubby Thought

Very Low-Calorie Diets (VLDL)

"The weight loss observed in patients given a liquid diet providing 420 kcal/day was not significantly greater than that observed in persons who consumed a liquid diet providing 800 kcal/day."

"This suggests that patients treated with VLCDs are either less compliant with the diet or sustain a greater decline in energy expenditure than those treated with LCDs." p. 1619

Williams Textbook of Endocrinology, 2011, 12th edition, Shlomo Melmed et al., Elsevier Saunders.

Reference cited: Foster et al. A Controlled Comparison of Three Very-Low-Calorie Diets: Effects on Weight, Body Composition, and Symptoms. Am J Clin Nutr., 1992, 55:811-817.

Chapter 9

Alaskan Cruise

September

Weight 9-11-11: 246.5 lbs.

LDL-P 1,097 (goal < 750)
LDL-C 57 (goal < 70)
Tubby Factor 70 (goal < 80)
Insulin resistance 68 (goal? < 27)
ApoB 63 (goal < 60)
Small LDL P 538 (goal? < 117)
LDL size 20.9 nm (goal > 20.8)
HDL-C 44 (goal > 40)
HDL-P 33.7 (goal > 35)
Triglyceride 65 (goal < 100)

(Lab done on August 27 in Orlando before the Alaskan cruise.) Later, I realized my glucose was out of control at this time as I had stopped Actos in May.

I flew first-class to Seattle with 50,000 frequent-flier miles. The Admiralty lounge was not available unless I went international first-class. I had a three-hour layover in Dallas. We arrived in Seattle too late to take the light-rail for $2.50 as it closes down five minutes after midnight.

Forty-dollar cab ride and we checked into a great room in the Westin as they upgraded us to a larger room on the forty-first floor facing Elliot Bay because of our platinum status.

Our friends showed us a new side of Seattle. We saw a show at the Triple Door, had breakfast at Turfs, and went to Julia's for a drag show. After two nights, we boarded our ship for Alaska.

The big news of the cruise was that we could not see Hubbard Glacier because of a hurricane. However, the replacement was excellent. We went to Tracy Arm Glacier and the fjords, which we had not seen before.

We flew home to Jensen Beach. I then drove my dog and I home in two nights and three days. After 1,600 miles of driving, I was quite concerned about my weight. To my surprise, my weight was 246.5 lbs. The next day it was 249.5 lbs., and the third day it was 249 lbs. Later, I realized this weight loss was due to stopping Actos in May.

This was great news. With virtually no exercise for six days after the cruise, I was the same weight as last month. I was 9 lbs. less than I was in January. I did this without hunger and with intermittent exercise. On the cruise I did try to walk the deck for 2 miles a day, and we took the stairs.

Why did my LDL-P go up? I am not certain. (I now suspect it is because my glucose was out of control) Why did my HDL-C go down? Clearly, it was because I had not been taking my Actos. Why did my insulin resistance number go up? Clearly, it was because I had not been taking my Actos.

Stopping Actos was a very big mistake as seen by my Hgb A1C going above 10. This was an important lesson for me. A very low-carbohydrate diet for a diabetic does not negate the need for medicine.

If I had lost 20 lbs., maybe I could get away with decreasing Actos. However, even when I was down to 200 lbs., I stayed on Actos 45 mg. Once a person is an insulin-resistant diabetic, it is important to stay on Actos.

I had stopped Actos on the advice of a low-carb guru who was trying to help me figure out why I wasn't losing more weight. Actos causes weight gain, but it causes peripheral-fat weight gain. It causes water-retention weight gain. Peripheral fat is not the bad fat. After I stopped the Actos, I noticed my abdomen became tense and full. My story is only one case study, but I do believe there are lessons to be learned.

Lipid instruction

Is diabetes a disease of glucose primarily or a disease of lipids? Actos made all the difference for my Hgb A1C and my insulin resistance despite the fact that my weight is 9 lbs. less than in January and while on a very low-carb diet.

This time I think my LDL-P went up because of my insulin resistance and not weight gain. Compare this to my results in March. My apoB was great at 63 with VAP calculation in August. This result is discordant with the LDL-P of 1,097 done at the same time by Liposcience lab. Unfortunately, I believe this discordance reflects that the VAP apoB is not as accurate as the LDL-P in tubby patients.

Another lesson is that a high-fat diet with alcohol consumption and niacin are not the main contributors to my HDL-C, the lack of Actos made a difference in HDL-C. However, if you use the HDL-P, which is probably more accurate, there is not much change.

Off Actos, I had the following changes in HDL types:

	May 2011	August 2011 (off Actos with Hgb A1C at 10)
Liposcience Lab		
HDL-C	61	44
HDL-P	35.7	33.7
Large HDL-P	7.5	1.5
HDL size	9.3	8.4
VAP LAB		
HDL 2		17 (goal > 10) large, buoyant, more protective
HDL 3		39 (goal > 30) small, dense, less protective
Apo A1	163	149 (goal > 118)

I wrote in my book *The Tubby Theory from Topeka* in January 2010 that HDL was a conundrum.

HDL still is a puzzle. It is for this reason I don't pay attention to the HDL ratios.

There is a large variance between the large HDL in Liposcience and in VAP. There is a general decrease in all the numbers since I stopped Actos. The HDL-C number would make me think there was a drastic drop in my HDL. The HDL-P number shows that my HDL change was not that drastic. I had about the same amount of HDL particles, they held less cholesterol and were smaller.

Bottom line: It's the LDL-P that is important. If the apoB, LDL-C, and Tubby Factor were the only parameters, I would have no idea that my particle was off due to the metabolic syndrome IR being very high.

The prior lipid studies look at HDL-C and LDL size.

Let's see some studies that have low fat versus low carb that use advanced lipid testing and concentrate on LDL-P. My lab this month shows that there is discordance as the metabolic syndrome gets worse. Why is the apoB different than the LDL-P? VAP uses a calculation for apoB rather than direct testing with immunoassay as Berkley Heart Lab does. However, in severe metabolic syndrome, there may be a distortion of the LDL particle that the immunoassay will read falsely low. Further research is needed to get to the bottom of this controversy.

Tubby Thought

Can You Eat 7 Calories/Pound a Day and Walk 5 Miles Every Day of Your Life to Maintain Your Weight?

"Treatment of Obesity obviously must lead to a negative energy balance, preferably through reducing food intake and increasing energy expenditure. Even though this strategy sounds simple in theory (according to the first law of thermodynamics), decades of advocating weight loss have failed to stop the obesity epidemic" (Dubnov-Raz and Berry, Medical Clinics of North America [September 2011], p. 940).

Weight Maintenance and the Reduced Obese

"A clue may be found when studying a 'rare' clinical subject: a reduced obese person who has succeeded in losing weight and maintaining the new body weight for more than a year. The National Weight Control Registry documented the metabolic and behavioral cost of maintaining a reduced obese state of maintaining a reduced obese state for more than 5 years."
Men 1225 kcal/d net after exercise
Women 918 kcal/d net after exercise p. 945
Dubnov-Raz and Berry
Medical Clinics of North America Sept. 2011

Caveat emptor:

There are 6,000 of the reduced obese that have succeeded by maintaining a substarvation diet. How many of the reduced obese failed due to the many compensatory mechanisms of the body to prevent starvation? Millions.

Low-calorie diets ultimately fail due to the reduced obese suffering from the Sponge Syndrome. They increase weight like a sponge. After my diet, I weighed 200 lbs. The NWCR suggests 7 cal/lb. $\times$ 200 = 1,400 calories a day. My 5 miles walking would burn not 500 calories but 300 calories due to the 42% reduction in my exercise metabolism. This is for maintenance!

Chapter 10

Orlando

October
Weight 10-7-11: 249 lbs.

I went to the Obesity Society (TOS) meeting in Orlando from 9-31-11 to 10-5-11. I learned a new term: reduced obese. As I have tried to explain that there are Tubbies and there are Twiggies and that each has their own calorie math, I found confirmation in Orlando.

A scientist said the first law of thermodynamics is in place and a calorie is still a calorie.

I asked the scientist about the gut microbes. He said that is an interesting area. I looked it up in George Bray's book, *A Guide to Obesity and the Metabolic Syndrome* (2011). He writes on page 72, "The kinds of microbes in the gut may affect body weight . . . and lean individuals possess more of the Bacteroidetes and the obese more of the Firmicutes (Ley et al. 2006)." Also on page 73, he writes, "A study in individuals with gastric bypass bariatric surgery showed that the bacterial colonization shifted towards the types of microbes seen in normal weight individuals and away from the obese (Zhang et al. 2009)."

The concept of leptin threshold was discussed at this meeting. Fat cells (adipocytes) make leptin. Leptin tells the brain how much fat there is in the body. The thin person has less fat and thus less leptin. The fat person has much more leptin. Thus it has been said that the fat person is leptin resistant. This is why injecting leptin into fat people does not make them lose weight. The scientist was saying we have to look at it differently. It is threshold, not resistance.

With significant weight loss, the leptin threshold will change, the brain puts us on a different EE, a more efficient energy expenditure, so that we don't lose more weight.

Diet and Exercise programs have and will fail because of *the reduced obese problem*. I will repeat the North American Clinics quote several times as I believe it is so important. Look at the people who have succeeded. The National Weight Control Registry has a list of 6,000 people who have succeeded.

In the Obesity Issue of Medical Clinics of North American Sept. 2011, on page 945, Dubnov-Raz and Berry write, "Both men and women (in the NWCR) consumed a low-fat diet (24%) and exercised to use 470 to 360 calories kcal/d, respectively. The net energy balance was 918 kcal/d for women and 1225 kcal/ for men. These reduced obese subjects ate an average of five meals a day and conducted a very regimented existence."

I went to the Obesity Society meeting in Orlando at the Marriott World Resort. I did very little exercise as I sat listening to the lectures. I had been eating a lot of nuts lately. Otherwise, I ate at the restaurants for five days. Breakfast at the grill in the first floor made my three eggs and bacon easy. Lunch was easy with the chef salad from the grill with three tubs of blue cheese dressing. Dinner worked out at the sports bar in the hotel. They had a happy hour. I had the fried chicken with buffalo sauce sandwich. I skipped the bun. I didn't drink any alcohol for the five days.

I am running 9 lbs. less than last January. My glucose is still high at 190-220 each morning.

I went to Onamia, Minnesota, this past week. Five days in a car touring around. I gained 6.5 lbs. I weighed in at 255.5. The autumn leaves were nice but nothing to compare to Vermont. Duluth was interesting. The effect of the Lake Superior on the weather was interesting. It snowed 53 inches in Duluth while it snowed 350 inches in the Upper Peninsula. I saw a Squarepants Sponge Bob statue in the Mall of America, and I realized that the reduced obese suffer from the Sponge Syndrome. They soak up calories like a sponge. I met two Minnesota Vikings Cheerleaders at the Mall of America. They asked me if I was a Vikings fan. I said I am now. Who says middle America is boring?

I joined the Fat Head group on Facebook to talk to people like me who believe in low-carb diet. I was welcomed, but my efforts to explain my position on statins did not go over well. I hope to be a bridge between lipidologists and low-carb fans.

I have read *The Cholesterol Myths* by Uffe Ravnskov, MD. I found his analysis of Ancel Keys Seven Nations Trial to be wonderful. I have *The Great Cholesterol Con* by Malcom Kendricks.

I had read chapter 6 entitled "Eat Whatever You Like. (Diet Has Nothing to Do with Heart Disease)." I think that high-fat diet with low-carb diet has nothing to do with heart disease in most people. However, I think someone like Tim Russert who continued to have high triglyceride and low HDL-C, after failing with statin and niacin and trilipex should have been tried on a very low-carb diet with 4,000 mg of fish oil.

I started reading *The Great Cholesterol Con* again. I saw that the date of publication was 2007. I wanted something more current and I found this site on Jimmy Moore

http://www.thelivinlowcarbshow.com/shownotes/271/dr-malcom-kendrick-debunks-the-great-cholesterol-con-episode-263
Dr. Malcolm Kendrick Debunks The Great Cholesterol Con (Episode 263) *http://www.thelivinlowcarbshow.com/*

This interview was June 18, 2009. There was little that I disagreed with. Malcolm Kendrick clearly states in the interview what is good about statins. He says for high risk men with heart disease it does have benefit.

I was also reading what Dr. Mike Eades thought of the Jupiter trail. He wrote that Crestor was good for people with a high sensitive c-reactive protein.

See Dr. Mike Eades article about Jupiter on *http://www.proteinpower.com/drmike/cardiovascular-disease/1853/*
The Blog of Michael R. Eades, MD » Truth versus hype in the Jupiter study *http://www.proteinpower.com/ www.proteinpower.com*

Actual quote from Dr. Eades's article: "Let's look at it in the best light possible. If we do, we find that a small group of unusual patients - those with low LDL-cholesterol AND high C-reactive protein - may slightly decrease their risk for all-cause mortality by taking a drug that costs them almost $1,300 per year and slightly increases their risk for developing diabetes. That's the best spin possible given the data from this study. Compare that to the spin the media is giving it."

That might seem like faint praise indeed but I suspect that since he wrote this article he may have read Dr. Allan Sniderman's analysis of Jupiter in Current Atherosclerosis Reports 2009, 11: 358-363. Dr. Sniderman points out the average LDL-C was 108, which is the twenty-fifth percentile for risk while the apoB was 109, which is the sixtieth percentile for men and the seventieth percentile for women for risk. The people in the Jupiter trial were not at low risk. The discordance between

LDL-C and apoB (the particles) showed that the study was done on high risk people and not low risk people. Older books that talk about cholesterol and LDL are out of date in their terminology. It has to be specified if they are talking about total cholesterol or LDL-C or LDL-P or apoB.

In people with metabolic syndrome there is usually a discordance between LDL-C and LDL-P. Very important to make this clear in your discussions.

Doctor Mercola writes, "I believe it (total cholesterol) should be about 200 or so."

"When you have a cholesterol of 150, it's too low, because cholesterol is an important element of your cell membranes and it's a precursor for steroid [hormones]. You need cholesterol . . . the HDL to total cholesterol should be greater than 25%."

http://mercola.fileburst.com/PDF/VideoTanscript-cholesterol-statin%20_1-21.pdf
mercola.fileburst.com/PDF/VideoTanscript-cholesterol-statin%20_1-21.pdffileburst.com
https://www.facebook.com/ajax/sharer/?s=99&appid=2309869772&p%5B0%5D=66
https://www.facebook.com/groups/57440891958/10150501464131959/
Some facts:

1. A new born baby has an LDL-C of 40. The brain grows very rapidly on this level of LDL-C.
2. People born with hypolipobetaproteinemia have LDL-C below 10-15 mg/l. They have no ill effects and have longevity.
3. Almost every cell in the body can make its own cholesterol.
4. The Jupiter trial took several thousand people down to an LDL-C average of 55 mg/dl. Many of the people went down to 35 mg/l. There were no ill effects. There was an increase in diabetes which we still don't understand, however most of these people were prediabetic before the study and many had metabolic syndrome. Based on the above facts I give statins. See Steinberg et al. 1979, Metabolic studies in an unusual case of asymptomatic familial hypobetalipoproteinemia. J Clin Invest, 64: 292-301

Tubby Thought

Aging Metabolism

"Older people have a lower metabolic expenditure than younger ones and as a rule lose weight more slowly since metabolic rates decline by approximately 2% per decade (about 100 kcal per decade) Lin et al. 2003" (George Bray, *A Guide to Obesity and the Metabolic Syndrome: Origins and Treatment* [CRC Press, 2011], p. 178).

Chapter II

Palm Desert, California

November
Weight 253.5 pounds

Despite my frequent travels, I find that the airlines and timeshares still take me to school. We like to fly out to our timeshare in Palm Springs a week before we fly across the Pacific. This breaks up a very long plane journey. The most difficult part of travel is the air travel. It is not for sissies. We made a reservation with Travelocity and chose a more expensive flight in order to fly direct nonstop from Kansas City to Los Angeles. We had printed out our itinerary, and it showed flight 775 leaving from MCI (KC) at 8:05 AM to LAX (LA) nonstop. The night before we flew, we tried to check in online with Frontier Airline. I found out our flight had been changed to 6:30 AM departure and we were changing planes in Denver before flying to LAX. Apparently, Travelocity should have contacted us, but the notice might have been lost in the spam filter. We woke up at 3:30 AM to drive seventy-five minutes to the airport. We arrived at LAX at 1:30 PM central time. We arrived at Westin Mission Hills at 4:00 PM central time. We traveled for twelve hours. The lesson I learned is, only make reservations with the airline directly or make certain Travelocity or Orbitz does contact you with changes. When they notify me of a change, I need to pay attention.

We are platinum members of the Starwood system of hotels and timeshares. On the hotel side, it has paid off royally. On the timeshare side, there are very few perks. We purchased a promotion plan with Mission Hills that would allow us to buy 70,000 points inexpensively. We checked in and told them we are platinum members. They put us in the worse "deluxe villa" with no view and poor location.

We are also platinum members in Diamond Resorts. They claim that they will steer us to the best locations in the resorts with a special concierge. That remains to be seen.

This is my third trip to the Palm Springs area. I love this area. We went to Roy's for a great happy hour. Drinks and appetizers for $5. Is America great or what? In an Irish pub, I had to buy bourbon and sweet vermouth in separate glasses and mix it myself. The euro is not kind to cocktails. In Canada, the cocktails are small. At Roy's, they made a wonderful Manhattan and Ahi roll for a total of $10.

We spent three nights at the SLS Hotel in Beverly Hills. It is in the Starwood collection of hotels, and we were upgraded to a big suite with a corner window. We ate at the Bazaar restaurant on the grounds. Very expensive. It was balanced by a trip to Pinky's hot dog stand. After a thirty-minute wait, we had wonderful hot dogs.

Tubby Thought

Rewrite All the Books on Obesity

"For instance, the recent discoveries in genetics have found that people differ in their perceptions of hunger and satiety on a genetic basis and that predisposed subgroups of the population may be particularly vulnerable to obesity in "obesogenic" societies with unlimited access to food. This notion must lead to a more open attitude toward obese people and a reduction in discrimination against them [*http://www.ncbi.nlm.nih.gov/pubmed/18971438* 123], it is clear that obesity cannot be considered as a consequence only of indolence or lack of will, as often thought in our societies. In the long term, we are confident that progress in genetics will help to develop useful diagnostic and predictive tests and design new treatments."

Curr Genomics. 2011 May; 12(3):169-79.
Genetics of Obesity: What have we Learned?
Choquet H, Meyre D.
Source: Ernest Gallo Clinic and Research Center, Department of Neurology, University of California, San Francisco, Emeryville, California 94608, USA.

Abstract
Candidate gene and genome-wide association studies have led to the discovery of nine loci involved in Mendelian forms of obesity and 58 loci contributing to polygenic obesity. These loci explain a small fraction of the heritability for obesity and many genes remain to be discovered. However, efforts in obesity gene identification greatly modified our understanding of this disorder. In this review, we propose an overlook of major lessons learned from 15 years of research in the field of genetics and obesity. We comment on the existence of the genetic continuum between monogenic and polygenic forms of obesity that pinpoints the role of genes involved in the central regulation of food intake and genetic predisposition to obesity. We explain how the identification of novel obesity predisposing genes has clarified unsuspected biological pathways involved in the control of energy balance that have helped to understand past human history and to explore causality in epidemiology. We provide evidence that obesity predisposing genes interact with the environment and influence the response to treatment relevant to disease prediction.

Chapter 12

Paul Gauguin Cruise to
Society Islands and Marquesas

December
Weight 256 pounds

The final data has come in for my book:

	12-9-11	12-18-07	1-10-2006	2-6-01
CAC	7.9	1.0	20	8.0

	12-6-2011	8-27-11	5-20-11	3-12-11	8-28-10
LDL-P	842	1,097	765	1,246	651

CIMT	right carotid	left carotid
12-6-11:	0.50 mm	0.59 mm
11-19-09:	0.52 mm	0.54 mm
7-29-08:	0.50 mm	0.58 mm

All the above were done on the same Philips iU22 ultrasound machine at Stormont Vail Medical Center and interpreted by the same physician.

6-1-07:   0.639 mm   0.743 mm

Above was done on ArterioVision.   Done at a lipid conference by specialists in the field.

I have been on a 60% fat diet for the last year. I have not lost weight. I have not gained weight. I have eaten on a cruise ship for ninety days in the last year.

The CIMT scores reflect the atheroma in the wall of my carotids. They did not change much from 2.5 years ago, and they are still much better than my first CIMT in June 2007.

My CAC is higher than it was in 2007 but still much better than 2006. All the CACs were done on different machines. This is the first time I had it done while in atrial fibrillation. This may make the most recent reading less accurate. I would maintain that keeping my CAC under 10 since 2001 by keeping my LDL-P around 750 is the significant fact. My systolic blood pressure has been well controlled with Ramipril. My diabetic control has been more erratic.

Aging alone will thicken the carotid wall and add some calcium to the wall of the coronary artery.

I had four LDL-P's done while on a very low-carbohydrate diet with less exercise than 2010 and without net weight gain or weight loss. I was on Crestor 5mg/d plus Endur-acin 1,000 mg and Lovaza 4,000 mg in 2010 and all of 2011. The first LDL-P of 1,246 after my first two months of a very low-carb diet was of concern. The explanation is not clear. I did a lot of long range driving in Scotland, Ireland, and America. This prolonged sedentary activity is my best explanation. I did very little exercise during these two months.

This is only one case study. I would propose that following the LDL-P, CAC, and CIMT is the best way to determine if your diet is working for you. Thin people die from heart attacks and strokes and sudden death. Follow your plaque.

Fourteen days on the Paul Gauguin in the South Pacific. At 4:00 PM, I would go to the tea/bar hour at the back of the eighth deck. I didn't have a veranda in my room, thus I would sit at the back of the deck bar and enjoy the late afternoon sun hanging over the sea. I would have a glass of Cabernet Sauvignon with the finger sandwiches. I would not eat the bread. Then I would move on from wine to a Manhattan to get into a relaxed South Seas mood. The desserts were superb, but I was able to resist them. I might take a little bit of some sweet morsel at rare moments. This was the best time of my day. I would have three eggs with bacon and sausage for breakfast until I discovered I could have minute steak with delicious béarnaise sauce. Lunch was typically the best meal of the day. I would make a salad with blue cheese dressing and then have two of the meat entrées and a glass of good red wine. The cheese selection was exceptional. The pastries on the Gauguin are probably among the best, if not the best on the high seas. Dinner was better than in most cruise lines. However, the two specialty restaurants on Oceania *Nautica* were better yet. The Paul Gauguin cruise is unique. However, it is for people who love to travel. I would advise Hawaii first to anyone.

I came back from the Paul Gauguin Cruise and had gained about 3.5 lbs. My weight was about the same as it was in January 2011 when I began my 60% fat diet. Future studies need to always screen for CIMT, CAC, and LDL-P. I did this for myself. My CAC this week cost $50. My CIMT cost $100 last week. CAC and CIMT with morning blood pressure monitoring and LDL-P blood testing are much more important in determining health than eating antioxidants, high fiber, low animal fat, and excising more than twenty minutes a day. Therapeutic lifestyle changes cannot compare to having an LDL-P of 750. Let's concentrate on what we know works. LDL-P of 750 works.

Secondarily, walk for twenty minutes, avoid being sedentary for long periods, and don't gain weight. I did not gain weight over the last year on a low-carb, high-fat, high-protein diet. This may not be the best for every genetic profile, but for the Tubbies of the world, it may be. Short-term weight loss with a low-calorie diet may be a bad thing if it makes you one of the reduced obese. About 95% of you will gain your weight back.

I don't have the solution for everyone, but I have maintained my weight this year with a high-fat diet, and I have not been hungry. I exercised less, and I was on a cruise ship for ninety days this year. This case study is simply a call to reexamine the data and open our minds to the fact that the present paradigm of fruits and vegetables and low fat may not be the best diet for people with the metabolic syndrome.

Math

250 lbs. × 10 kcal = 2,500 kcal/day to maintain weight
250 lbs. × 7 kcal = 1,750

My crude resting metabolism test showed I burned 1,750 calories a day

breakfast:

3 eggs, 300 calories
3 strips of bacon, 150 calories

lunch:

4 oz. cold cuts, 400 calories
2 oz. of cheese, 150 calories
1tbs. mayonnaise, 100 calories

dinner:

10 oz. fillet, 1,000 calories
2 tbs. salad blue cheese dressing, 150 calories
3 oz. alcohol, 300 calories

Total: 2,450 calories a day

Walking 2 miles a day $= 200$ calories a day
200 calories $\times 0.42\% = 84$ calories
$200 - 84 = 116$ calories burned with exercise

Net calories a day: $2,450 - 116 = 2,334$

$2,500 - 2,334 = 166$ calories deficit

$166 \times 30 = 3980$ calorie deficit a month

3,500 calories to burn 1 lb. of fat

I should lose a little more than a pound a month per month. However, since I am one of the reduced obese do I need to eat 7 cal/lb. or 1,750 cal/day as per the NWCR which is supported by the resting metabolism test that showed I burn 1,750 calories a day without exercise?

1,750 calories − 116 calories = 1,534 net calories to maintain 250 lbs.
I eat 2,450 calories a day with no hunger
2,450 − 1,534 = 916 excess calories a day
916 calories × 4 days = 3,664 calories.
I should gain 1 lb. every four days on the very low-carbohydrate diet outlined above.

I know I have eaten at least 2,450 calories a day in 2011.
When I drove the car on trips or flew in an airplane, I did not do any exercise.
On cruises I probably walked 3-4 miles a day most of the time but not on the River cruise in Europe. Thus an average of 2 miles walking a day for the year is a fair estimate.

Since I was 258 lbs. when I started the diet and 258 lbs. when I finished the diet, I believe either calorie calculation was wrong. As a diabetic, eating 20-40 g of carbohydrate a day changes the dynamic of counting calories as carb drives insulin drives fat accumulation. Perhaps the 30 g of protein at each of the three meals also drives the metabolism more.

This is one case study. It begs the question of better trials in the future with LDL-P, CAC, CIMT measurement in participants that remain on the 20-40 g of carbohydrate all year long.

January 2012 End of Case Study: 1-4-11 to 1-3-12

End Points of Case Study

End Point One: LDL-P

8-28-10	3-12-11	5-20-11	8-27-11	12-5-11
651	1246	765	1097	842

End Point Two: Coronary Calcium Score (CAC)

	2-6-01	1-10-06	12-18-07	12-9-11
CAC	8.0	20	1.0	7.9

End Point Three: Carotid Intimal Medial Thickness (CIMT)

CIMT	6-1-07	7-29-08	11-19-09	12-06-11
right:	0.639	0.50	0.52	0.50
left:	0.743	0.58	0.54	0.59

End Point Four: Weight:

Jan. 3, 2011	256 pounds
Jan. 3-12	256 pounds

End Point Five: Hgb A1C

8-28-10	3-12-11	5-20-11	8-27-11	12-5-11
8.7	8.2	7.7	10.3	9.5

I visited my Jensen beach physician. Last Aug. 23, 2011, he had my weight at 249 lbs. after I had stopped my Actos in May. However, my Hgb A1C had shot up to 10.1. I immediately went back on my Actos 45 and increased my metformin back to 2,000 mg a day. About four months later, I weighed 256 lbs. I had lost weight off Actos but gained weight back since I started Actos again. Unfortunately, my Hgb A1C has only gone down to 9.5.

The reason I began the low-carbohydrate diet last January was because I was gaining 1.5 lbs. per month despite two to three hours of exercise a day. My Hgb A1C was also creeping up and reached 8.7. On the low-carbohydrate diet my Hgb A1C decreased to 8.2 and then 7.7 after a forty-five-day cruise. I was not losing weight on the low-carb diet. A low-carb guru suggested I stop Actos as that might be preventing my weight loss. I stopped Actos in May. I weighed 257 lbs. I lost 8 lbs. off Actos and I gained 7 lbs. back on Actos. The peripheral weight I gained from Actos is peripheral weight and not the toxic central obesity. Thus, theoretically the extra weight did not contribute to my Hgb A1C remaining relatively high at 9.5 despite getting back to Actos 45 mg and increasing my metformin from 1,000 mg to 2,000. What was the exercise variable. Insulin resistance is treated by Actos, metformin and especially a lot of exercise.

The Exercise Confounding Co-Variables:

1. On the forty-five-day cruise, I always took the stairs, and I did a good amount of walking every day after each meal. I also was lifting weights.
2. The twenty-one-day European cruise was not so good. The walking area on the roof of the *Prestige* was dismantled for most of the voyage. No weight lifting. I purchased the Silver collection which increased my alcohol intake to the highest point of my life for two weeks.
3. After my fourteen-day Paul Gauguin Cruise I again had unlimited alcohol, but I exercised much more than the European cruise but not as much as the forty-five-day cruise. Not very scientific but the best I can do.

Conclusions:

1. I finally stopped gaining weight by going on a low-carbohydrate diet.
2. The low-carbohydrate did not obviate the needs for diabetic medications.
3. Despite eating 60% fat in my diet, my LDL-P ended at an excellent level.
4. My CIMT showed no increase in atheroma my carotids.
5. My CAC did not show an increase from my first CAC. There was some increase from a prior CAC but different machines were used, and this last time I was in atrial fibrillation when the study was done.

Final advanced lipid test done on 12-28-2011 by Berkeley Heart Lab

Total Cholesterol 146
LDL-C 79
HDL-C 53
Triglycerides 70
Tubby Factor 93
Apo B 62
Lp-PLAC2 162
CRPhs 0.7
Lp(a) 38

The apoB is the one number that is most significant. It measures all the atherogenic particles except Lp(a). After a year of eating 60% fat, I have an excellent apoB.

At the Orlando battle, people said I have good genes. I am a diabetic with ApoE genotype 3/4, a KIF6 of Trp/Arg and an LPA-Aspirin genotype of Ile/Ile and have always had a high Lp(a). None of that information suggests I have good genes.

In the sixties and the seventies when the country decided low-fat diets were healthy, I believe a big mistake was made in regards to diabetics and patients with metabolic syndrome. I hope the Tubbies in America will try to reevaluate themselves with:

1. CAC
2. CIMT
3. LDL-P

(while staying on a low-carb diet of 20-40 g a day and walking at least eight to twenty minutes a day.)

I believe my yearlong case study makes a very strong argument for such an effort.

Travelogue 2011

1. Aviemore and the Cairngorms, Scotland (1-15-11 to 1-23-11)
   Scottish breakfast is a good source of protein and fat. Stay away from the scones, which I don't care for.
2. Dublin, Ireland (1-22-11 to 1-26-11)
   Tour of the Guinness Brewery provides a great view and a beer. The carb content of 17 g in a Guinness Beer destroyed my low-carb diet. We spent five days at the Westin. While in Ireland the government collapsed. I asked locals who was running the government. They did not know. They seemed resigned. Before when times were bad, they had a pint at the local pub. Now they can't even afford to do that.
3. Athlone, Ireland (1-27-11 to 2-1-11)
   We visited the oldest pub in Ireland. It was one of those times to break the low-carb diet with a Guinness. We spent five days at the Sheraton.
4. Wyndham Bonnet Creek Resort, Florida (2-13-11 to 2-19-11)
   A timeshare allows the low-carb dieter to roast a turkey in their suite.

5. Jensen Beach, Henderson Island, Florida (2-19-11 to 3-5-11)
   We stayed at the Vistana timeshare for thirteen days. The kitchen allows us to make steaks and eat salads for a reasonable price.
6. W New Orleans Hotel, Louisiana (3-6-11 to 3-11-11)
   I avoided the Bananas Foster by eating many oysters and drinking classic gin martinis during Mardi Gras.
7. Hyatt Regency Lost Pines Resort and Spa, Texas (3-11-11 to 3-13-11)
   This NLA conference provided several "healthy" meals. However, they don't believe in low-carb, high-fat diets. I had three boiled eggs for breakfast with coffee. Nice place outside of Austin, Texas.
8. Westin Mission Hills Villas (3-19-11 to 3-24-11)
   Our Starwood timeshare kitchen allows me to cook eggs, bacon, hamburgers, chicken, and steaks. We do love the happy hour in the Palm Springs area, especially the Falls.
9. W Hong Kong Hotel 3-25-11
   Peking duck at the Spring Deer restaurant was great. McDonald's was available. I didn't eat the buns. I did break the diet for dim sum.
10. Oceania Cruise on the Nautica (3-26-11 to 5-10-11)
    We cruised for forty-five days from Hong Kong to Athens during Arab Spring. We missed Cairo as a result. A cruise ship is a great place for a low-carb diet.
11. Hue, Thua Thien, Hue Province, Vietnam (3-29-11)
    We docked at Da Nang. The buffet lunch in Vietnam was better food than what we got in China.
12. Ho Chi Minh City, Vietnam (4-1-11 to 4-2-11)
    The locals call it Saigon. Fifty motor vehicle deaths every day. Vietnam has the fastest-growing economy in the world. We purchased a lacquer painting of cherry blossoms and mailed it home.
13. Singapore (4-3-11 to 4-3-11)
    This was the biggest disappointment of the trip. I heard Christmas is very nice here.
14. Phuket, Thailand (4-5-11)
    We took a boat tour of the national park, which is one of the wonders of the world. We did not eat in Thailand.
15. Yangon (Rangoon), Myanmar (1-7-11 to 1-9-11)
    This is the place to buy gems. Our Internet was closed down because of the Arab Spring. The government switched from military to civilian, but the locals could not tell us anything about it. From our ship in a remote port, I could see seven pagodas across the countryside. The buffets in Burma were as good as in Saigon. Shwedagon Pagoda was the most impressive among many impressive pagodas and statues of Buddhas. Burma is known for its tapestries. We purchased a beautiful one at the market. They do negotiate to at least 50% of the initial price.

16. Kochi, Kerala, India (4-13-11)

    Cochin was a big surprise. The Chinese fishing nets were a reminder of the days when this was a major port of the ancient world. I never ate in India. I think beer is safe to drink anywhere in the world. However, I try to avoid beer on my low-carb diet. There is a Christian church here that predates Vasco da Gama!

17. Mumbai (Bombay), Maharashtra, India (4-13-11)

    I went to the Elephanta Ruins. There are five nuclear power plants surrounding Bombay. Our flight to Japan had been rerouted to Hong Kong because of the nuclear meltdown in Japan. Carbohydrates are a major threat to Indians. Despite a vegetarian diet, they are very prone to metabolic syndrome if their waist is more than thirty-five inches.

18. Muscat, Oman (4-18-11)

    We landed at Port Qaboos. There is a big fish market there. I did not eat here. Hummus is one of my loves, which I avoid as much as possible. Lamb is big in the Middle East. A rack of lamb makes being on a low-carb diet very easy. The Sultan Qaboos Grand Mosque was impressive.

19. Dubai, United Arab Emirates (4-19-11 to 4-20-11)

    This was a disappointment. About 90% of the people are workers who can never become citizens. The buildings are mostly empty. We had high tea at the sail building. For $100 the food was only fair. I wish I had taken the day tour to Abu Dhabi to see the Sheikh Zayed Grand Mosque instead of the high tea.

20. Fujairah, UAE (4-22-11)

    Some folks took the mountain desert tour here. Not much out there. We spent the day at an Internet shop. The Internet on the ship was very expensive and very slow. On the dock, I found a duty-free shop that sold me a bottle of jungle rum, vodka, and cognac for only $5 total. We enjoyed many sunsets with a cocktail on our deck.

21. Port Sultan Qaboos, Oman (4-23-11)

    The mosque here is worth seeing. This country is considered politically stable in this time of Arab Spring. The sultan of Omar made 50,000 jobs in the army after a demonstration from the people. He is a very mysterious person. Nothing is known of his personal life by the locals.

22. Salalah, Oman (4-25-11)

    I saw frankincense trees in the desert. I love stuffed grapes leaves. I didn't eat any here.

23. Gulf of Amen and Red Sea (4-26-11 to 4-29-11)

    The Nautica fought off a pirate attack a few years ago. The captain gave a great slide show about it. We had fire hoses at the ready on the deck. We also had four Israel security guards on board. Guns were not allowed on ship, but the captain had fended off the prior attack with ultrasonic wave machine. After hearing the talk, it seems a few guns would keep the pirates away. The pirates are angry about their fishing rights being abused. It is a big business. Apparently, the pirates use their booty to buy a mind-altering leaf from Kenya. I never got a chance to try the leaf. We cruised the Red Sea for three days. The best days on a cruise were the days at sea.

24. Aqaba, Jordan (4-30-11)

    We took the day tour to Petra. I was amazed by its beauty but sad to see little control of the crowds crawling over the ruins.

25. Luxor, Nile River Valley, Egypt (5-1-11 to 5-2-11)

    This was the highlight of the tour for me after Petra. I could not believe the excellent condition of the murals in the tombs. Wonderful. No crowds because of Arab Spring.

    We had lunch here, and I did get good hummus. Osama Bid Laden was killed at 1:00 AM local time. We learned about it the next morning.

26. Safaga, Red Sea, and Sinai (5-1-11 to 5-2-11)

    This is the port our ship was at. Some folks stayed the night a Luxor to watch the temples' light show. It was an extra expense but probably worth it.

27. Sharm El Sheikh, South Sinai, Egypt 5-3-11

    This was where I saw the most colorful coral I have ever seen while snorkeling. Shark attacks have occurred here. While shopping in this town, two Arabs asked my wife if she knew about Osama Bin Laden. She said they did not seem happy. Osama Bid Laden had been buried in the North Arabian Sea

28. Suez Canal, Egypt 5-4-11

    There is a monument to the AK-47 here.

29. Jerusalem, Israel (5-5-11 to 5-6-11) 5-4-11.

30. Haifa, Israel (5-7-11)

    We were diverted from Cairo because of the Arab Spring to a third night in Israel. I was happy because I was given a great orientation of the country from the Golan Heights to the south Dead Sea. Floating in the Dead Sea made seventy-year-olds act like kids. One couple left the cruise for an overnight flight to Cairo to see the pyramids. They had no trouble.

31. Ephesus, Izmir Province, Egypt (Kusadasi) (5-9-11)

    The ruins here are in good shape. I purchased a nice leather jacket here. We had the mint tea while shopping.

32. Athens, Greece (5-10-11 to 5-13-11)

    We left the ship here and spent two nights at the Grand Bretagne Hotel through Starwood points—20,000 points for two nights as it was the low season. They upgraded our room, and we had valet service. The first thing we did with the valet service was try to figure out what to do with the service. We did the obligatory nighttime dinner at the top of the hotel to see the Parthenon light up at night, but the real special event was smelling the tear gas from our window as the Greeks rioted in the plaza in front of us. It was all about the Greeks financial meltdown

33. Sheraton New York Hotel and Towers (5-18-11 to 5-23-11)
     Five nights with Starpoints gave me an upgrade to a large room with a view. I
     came to NYC for the National Lipid Association meeting. I met Atkins author
     Eric Westman. We ate meat at a place with a mechanical bull ride across from
     the skating rink. Only in NYC.

34. Ka'anapali Beach Club, Maui, Hawaii (5-29-11 to 6-10-11)
     This is a Diamond timeshare we have. I snorkeled off the beach in front of my
     timeshare and swam with a five-foot Hawaiian green turtle for ten minutes.
     There are so many turtles that many people want to take them off the
     endangered species list. Barefoot wine was only $5 in Walmart. Best bargain in
     Hawaii. Carb alert. I avoided the wonderful fruit and smoothies. This is not an
     easy diet sometimes.

35. St. Regis Princeville Resort, Princeville, Kauai (6-10-11 to 6-12-11)
     With our Starwood points and our platinum status, we got the best upgrade
     I have ever experienced. They gave us a junior suite with valet, overlooking
     Hanalei Bay. This may be best the most beautiful spot in the world. No kitchen
     here, but there was a sword ceremony to open a champagne bottle during
     happy hour on the veranda. I purchased a Bubba's Hamburger shirt for $10.
     This gave me free refills of soda. I ate at Bubba's about four times. The triple
     burger is perfect for the low-carb diet if you don't eat the bun.

36. The Point at Poipu, Kauai, Hawaii (6-12-11 to 6-25-11)
     On this trip we became platinum members in the Diamond club. To reward us,
     they gave us one of the nicest rooms at the Point. We had the view of the rock
     that Harrison Ford jumped off in Seven Days, Six Nights. Lots of young adults
     were making the jump. This is the garden island. There is a great trail along the
     coast here with many green turtles seen on the beach.

37. Hotel Pulitzer, Amsterdam, Noord-Holland, the Netherlands (6-30-11 to
     7-2-11)
     Platinum status in the Starwood point system again gave us a free upgrade to a
     large suite. I love the old buildings in Europe. Over the years I have eaten twice
     at Kantjil in Amsterdam. It reminds me of the colonial connection of Holland
     and Indonesia. Good food as well. I avoided the rice.

38. Viking river cruise on the *Prestige* (7-2-11 to 7-16-11)
     We cruised from Amsterdam to Budapest on this ship. A river cruise is very
     different from an ocean cruise. I grew up in NYC and like the superlatives. I like
     the big ocean ships. The food on the *Prestige* was good but not as good as the
     specialty restaurants on Oceania. There is little entertainment on a riverboat.
     The Silver Beverage Package made up for the lack of entertainment—unlimited
     wine and liquor for $300 per person. I wanted to drink the better wines of the
     different countries we cruised by. We made money on the deal.

39. Kinderdijk, Zuid-Holland, the Netherlands (7-3-11)

First day of cruise: Windmills. This World Heritage site is everything you expect from Holland. Windmills and the centuries old struggle against the sea.

40. Cologne, North Rhine-Westphalia (7-4-11)
Second day of cruise: Cathedral. The cathedral here was the tallest building in Europe till the Eiffel Tower was built. German wine of the day, Dornfelder, trocken.

41. Kobenz, Rhineland–Palatinate (7-5-1)
Third day of cruise: Castle. There are 1,000 types of sausages in Germany. This, with a wonderful variety of cheese, is why the Germans offer the best breakfasts in the world.

42. Miltenberg, Germany (7-6-11) Fourth day of cruise: Medieval town from AD1200.

43. Wurzburg, Romantic Road, Germany (7-7-11). Bishops Palace or the Wurzburg Residence is on the UNESCO World Heritage list. As a teenager, I was disappointed in the Hall of Mirrors at Versailles. I expected so much more. I found it forty years later in this marvelous Baroque palace. No disappointment here. It is grand! There is a ceiling fresco by G. B. Tiepolo above a three-story staircase (Treppenhaus), which is one of the great pieces of art of the world. The fresco measures about 7,300 square feet. The Sistine Chapel ceiling fresco is about 1,700 square feet.

44. Bamberg, Bavaria, Germany (7-8-11)
There are 300 breweries in Franconia, which is part of Bavaria.

45. Nuremburg, Germany (7-9-11)
A big surprise was the Congress Hall and stadium of the Nazi's that was built to have 400,000 seats–the ruins of the Third Reich.

46. Regensburg, Bavaria, Germany (7-10-11)
Oskar Schindler lived here in obscurity after the war.

47. Passau, Bayerischer Wald, Germany (7-11-11)
The organ at St. Stephens Cathedral is the second largest in the world. The largest is in Los Angeles. I was not impressed by the concert. The church is always covered by construction curtains. The inside is beautiful.

48. Melk, Danube Valley, Austria (7-12-11)
The Marble Hall and Library at the Babenberger castle is worth the visit.

49. Durnstein, Danube Valley (7-12-11)
This is a beautiful area.

50. Vienna, Austria (7-13-11)
Vienna, Budapest, and Bucharest do not disappoint, but Budapest is the most beautiful. Vienna, however, is a major challenge to a low-carbohydrate diet. I did break my diet for some cake and hot chocolate at Demel.

51. Bratislavia, Slovakia (7-14-11)
What a great little town, halfway between London and Istanbul.

52. Budapest, Hungary (7-15-11 to 7-16-11)

This is the jewel of the Danube. The lights at night from the river are sensational.

53. Boarded the viking *Prima Dona* to complete the voyage to Bucharest

    The *Prestige* was a brand-new ship. It had large thin-screen TVs with a library of movies to watch. The Internet on the *Prestige* was poor, but it completely vanished on the *Prima Dona*. Cruise lines and hotels need to make Internet fast and free if they want the next generation as their clients.

54. Kalocza, Hungary (7-17-11)

    To my surprise, I really enjoyed the horse show here. The cowboys in dresses did things with horses I had never seen at any rodeos out West.

55. Vukovar, Croatia (7-18-11)

    Poignant ruin of the water tower was from the attack by the Serbians.

56. Osijek, Croatia (7-18-11)

    The best beer in Eastern Europe is from Croatia.

57. Belgrade, Serbia (7-19-11)

    There is still damage from USA and NATO bombs here.

58. Iron Gate on the Danube River (7-20-11)

    The narrowest part of the Danube.

59. Viminacium, Serbia (7-20-11)

    A Roman ruins with a great future.

60. Veliko, Turnovo, Serbia (7-21-11)

    A fortress to hold off the invading Turks

61. Arbanasi, Serbia (7-21-11)

    Rose oil exporter.

62. Belogradchik Fortress (7-22-11)

    My favorite fortress.

63. Bucharest, Romania (7-23-11)

    The second-largest administrative building in the world is made of material from Romania.

64. Jensen Beach (7-7-11 to 7-11-11)

    We moved into our new condo on the beach.

65. Harborside Resort, Atlantis, Nassau (7-11-13 to 7-20-11)

    We snorkeled off Gilligan's Island. Nice coral.

66. Westin Seattle, Washington (8-31-11 to 9-3-11)

    I was disappointed in the buffets at Ivars. I don't think fish makes for good buffet.

67. Holland-American Cruise to Alaska (9-3-11 to 9-10-11)

    I did not like the layout of the Statendam. It seemed crowded and claustrophobic. The specialty restaurants were disappointing. The free Italian one was nothing special, and we had to pay $10 each for lunch at the Pinnacle. The fillet here was superior to what we ate in the main dining room.

68. Juneau, Alaska

The Mendenhall Glacier is getting smaller and dirtier.

69. Sitka, Alaska
   A pretty harbor, but after the Russian Orthodox Church, there really is nothing here. I advise folks to go out on whale expeditions.

70. Kitchacan, Alaska
   Friends had fun on the ship's city tour. I would suggest looking for whales if your budget can afford it.

71. Tracy Arm Glacier
   There was a hurricane that caused the captain to cancel the visit to Hubbard Glacier. The replacement of fjords and glaciers of Tracy Arm was almost as good.

72. Victoria, Canada
   The Jones Act requires that the ship stop in one foreign port before going back to Seattle. We had time to visit the famous hotel.

73. Orlando, Florida (9-30-11 to 10-5-11)
   World Center at Marriott for the Obesity Society meeting.

74. Itazys Resort, Viz Onamia, Minnesota (10-8-11 to 10-15-11)
   Mall of America, Duluth and Arrowhead

75. Westin Desert Willow, Palm Desert, California (11-11-11 to 11-14-11)
   Great place for happy hours.

76. SLS Hotel, LA, California (11-15-11 to 11-19-11)
   Very nice. Beverly Hills was full of thin well-dressed people.

77. Gaughin cruise in fourteen days (11-19-11 to 12-3-11)

78. Papeete
   The place has 170,000 people. You don't want to stay here. That's enormous for French Polynesia. More people fly into Hawaii in one day than fly into French Polynesia all year.

79. Fakarava
   A large atoll. You don't know what you have not missed until you have been to one. Good for the compulsive traveler.

80. Fatu Hiva, Manavave, Marquesas
   Many conservative people succumbed to the urge to get a tattoo here.

81. Hiva Oa
   Paul Gauguin museum. He attempted suicide here in Paradise. I also felt as if I spent two years here during the two-week cruise. Just kidding. It was wonderful for this tubby traveler.

82. Nuku Hiva (The photo on the cover of this book is from this island)
   This was called Madison Island when an American took it over. Amazing history! President Madison made him give it back. Herman Melville jumped ship here. Survivor series was here. The beach had such vicious biting flies that the contestants had to spend most of their time on a boat.

83. Taha

There was a private island here that was absolutely gorgeous.

I went on a drift snorkel tour here. A combination adventure ride with spectacular coral and fish.

84. Bora-Bora

The best manta ray interaction and the best snorkel experience I had in my life.

The guide said they take the Paul Gauguin tourists to a special coral garden. A recent cyclone destroyed much coral. I would advise newlyweds not to go to Bora-Bora unless they scuba dive. Good place to buy her a pearl.

85. Huahine

This may be the most beautiful island.

86. Moorea

Probably the place to stay at during September and October as the whales are here at that time.

There was a Club Med here. It closed in 2008. There were several places that died in French Polynesia at that time. The new Marlon Brando resort will be the place to go if you win the lottery.

87. Jensen Beach (12-19-11 to 1-5-12)

Christmas with family on the beach.

God bless America.

Personal Information	Sex: M	Date Drawn: 09/26/2009
Patient Name: EDWARDS,BRIAN	Age: 57	Date Tested: 09/29/2009
Account: TRADE SHOW VALIDATION	DOB: 12/27/1951	Accession: 6749700
Physician:	Client No: 101	Patient ID: 1347884

Cumulative Results

VAP Test Results	07/22/08	05/06/09
Total LDL	66	72
LDL-R (Real LDL)	48	55
Lp(a)	13.0	11
IDL	5	5
Total HDL	55	53
HDL_2	11	11
HDL_3	44	42
Total VLDL	14	18
$VLDL_{1+2}$	4.9	7.3
$VLDL_3$	9	10
Total Cholesterol	135	142
Triglycerides	60	103
Non-HDL Cholesterol	80	89
$Apo\ B_{100}$	64	65
Apo AI		154
$Apo\ B_{100}$/AI ratio		0.42

VAP Cholesterol Test

Patient Name: EDWARDS,BRIAN	Age: 57	Date Tested: 09/29/2009
Account: TRADE SHOW VALIDATION	DOB: 12/27/1951	Accession: 6749700
Physician:	Client No: 101	Patient ID: 1347884

Direct-Measured Cholesterol Panel	Actual	Desirable	Risk Low High	Description
Total LDL	55	<130 mg/dL		LDL-R + Lp(a) + IDL
LDL-R (Real LDL)	39	<100 mg/dL		Total LDL minus Lp(a) and IDL
Lp(a)	12	<10 mg/dL		More atherogenic than LDL
IDL	4	<20 mg/dL		More atherogenic than LDL
Total HDL	48	≥ 40 mg/dL		$HDL_2 + HDL_3$
HDL_2	12	>10 mg/dL		Large Buoyant, more protective
HDL_3	37	>30 mg/dL		Small Dense, less protective
Total VLDL	14	<30 mg/dL		$VLDL_{1+2} + VLDL_3$
$VLDL_{1+2}$	5.1	<20 mg/dL		Buoyant VLDL, less risk
$VLDL_3$	9	<10 mg/dL		Dense VLDL, more risk
Total Cholesterol	117	<200 mg/dL		LDL + HDL + VLDL

Secondary and Emerging Risk Factors	Actual	Desirable	Risk Low High	Description
Triglycerides	58	<150 mg/dL		Linked to increased risk for CHD
Non-HDL Cholesterol	68	<160 mg/dL		LDL + VLDL
Remnant Lipoproteins	13	<30 mg/dL		$IDL + VLDL_3$
Lp(a)	12	<10 mg/dL		More atherogenic than LDL
LDL Density (Pattern)	A	A		B: more risk; A/B intermediate risk; A: less risk

LDL Subclasses (mg/dL) LDL_4=6.8, LDL_3=19.7, LDL_2=9.1, LDL_1=3.1 LDL_{4+3} small, dense. LDL_{2+1} large, buoyant

VAP Derived Apolipoproteins	Actual	Desirable	Risk Low High	Description
$Apo\ B_{100}$	53	<109 mg/dL		Sum atherogenic lipoprotein particles
Apo AI	140	>118 mg/dL		Sum anti-atherogenic lipoprotein particles
$Apo\ B_{100}$/AI ratio	0.38	<0.92		Low ratio indicates lower risk

The VAP Cholesterol Test

Personal Information	Sex: M	Date Collected: 02/20/10
Patient Name: EDWARDS,BRIAN	Age: 58	Date Received: 02/23/10
Account: TRADE SHOW VALIDATION	DOB: 12/27/1951	Date Reported: 02/23/10
Physician:	Client No: 0518	Accession: 7032621

Cumulative Results

VAP Test Results	07/22/08	05/06/09	09/29/09	02/23/10
Total LDL	66	72	55	42
LDL-R (Real LDL)	48	55	39	27
Lp(a)	13.0	11	12	11
IDL	5	5	4	4
Total HDL	55	53	48	40
HDL$_2$	11	11	12	9
HDL$_3$	44	42	37	32
Total VLDL	14	18	14	14
VLDL$_{1+2}$	4.9	7.3	5.1	5.2
VLDL$_3$	9	10	9	9
Total Cholesterol	135	142	117	97
Triglycerides	60	103	58	62
Non-HDL Cholesterol	80	89	68	57
Apo B$_{100}$	64	65	53	48
Apo AI		154	140	126
Apo B$_{100}$/AI ratio		0.42	0.38	0.38

Cholesterol Test

Account: TRADE SHOW VALIDATION	DOB: 12/27/1951	Date Reported: 02/23/10
Physician:	Client No: 0518	Accession: 7032621

Direct-Measured Cholesterol Panel	Actual	Desirable	Risk Low	Risk High	Description
Total LDL	42	<130 mg/dL	▼		LDL-R + Lp(a) + IDL
LDL-R (Real LDL)	27	<100 mg/dL	▼		Total LDL minus Lp(a) and IDL
Lp(a)	11	<10 mg/dL		▼	More atherogenic than LDL
IDL	4	<20 mg/dL	▼		More atherogenic than LDL
Total HDL	40	≥ 40 mg/dL	▼		HDL$_2$ + HDL$_3$
HDL$_2$	9	>10 mg/dL		▼	Large Buoyant, more protective
HDL$_3$	32	>30 mg/dL	▼		Small Dense, less protective
Total VLDL	14	<30 mg/dL	▼		VLDL$_{1+2}$ + VLDL$_3$
VLDL$_{1+2}$	5.2	<20 mg/dL	▼		Buoyant VLDL, less risk
VLDL$_3$	9	<10 mg/dL	▼		Dense VLDL, more risk
Total Cholesterol	97	<200 mg/dL	▼		LDL + HDL + VLDL

Secondary and Emerging Risk Factors	Actual	Desirable	Risk Low	Risk High	Description
Triglycerides	62	<150 mg/dL	▼		Linked to increased risk for CHD
Non-HDL Cholesterol	57	<160 mg/dL	▼		LDL + VLDL
Remnant Lipoproteins	13	<30 mg/dL	▼		IDL + VLDL$_3$
Lp(a)	11	<10 mg/dL		▼	More atherogenic than LDL
LDL Density (Pattern)	A	A	▼		B: more risk; A/B intermediate risk; A: less risk

LDL Subclasses (mg/dL) LDL$_4$=6.4, LDL$_3$=14.8, LDL$_2$=5.0, LDL$_1$=0.9   LDL$_{4+3}$ small, dense. LDL$_{2+1}$ large, buoyant

VAP Derived Apolipoproteins	Actual	Desirable	Risk Low	Risk High	Description
Apo B$_{100}$	48	<109 mg/dL	▼		Sum atherogenic lipoprotein particles
Apo AI	126	>118 mg/dL	▼		Sum anti-atherogenic lipoprotein particles
Apo B$_{100}$/AI ratio	0.38	<0.92	▼		Low ratio indicates lower risk

Date Collected	Date Received	Report Date and Time	Requisition Number	Fasting Status
02/20/2010	02/23/2010	02/24/2010 01:03	16015077	FASTING

PARTICLE CONCENTRATION AND SIZE

LDL and HDL Particles		Lower CVD Risk				Higher CVD Risk
		Percentile in Reference Population[3]				
HDL-P (total)	μmol/L 28.3	high	75th 34.9	50th	25th 26.7	low
SMALL LDL-P	nmol/L 440	low	25th 117	50th	75th 839	high
LDL SIZE	nm 20.4	Large (Pattern A) 23.0	20.6	20.5	Small (Pattern B)	19.0

Small LDL-P and LDL Size are associated with CVD risk, but not after LDL-P is taken into account.

Lipoprotein Markers Associated with Insulin Resistance and Diabetes Risk[1,2]		Insulin Sensitive				Insulin Resistant
		Percentile in Reference Population[3]				
LARGE VLDL-P	nmol/L 1.5	low	25th 0.9	50th	75th 6.9	high
SMALL LDL-P	nmol/L 440	low	25th 117	50th	75th 839	high
LARGE HDL-P	μmol/L 4.3	high	75th 7.3	50th	25th 3.1	low
VLDL SIZE	nm 47.4	small	25th 42.4	50th	75th 52.6	large
LDL SIZE	nm 20.4	large	75th 21.2	50th	25th 20.4	small
HDL SIZE	nm 9.3	large	75th 9.6	50th	25th 8.9	small

Insulin Resistance Score

LP-IR SCORE**	0-100 42	insulin sensitive	25th 27	50th	75th 63	insulin resistant

Date Collected	Date Received	Report Date and Time	Requisition Number	Fasting Status
02/20/2010	02/23/2010	02/24/2010 01:03	16015077	FASTING

NMR LipoProfile® test

Reference Range[1]

	nmol/L	Low	Moderate	Borderline-High	High	Very High
		Percentile[1]	20th	50th	80th	95th
LDL-P (LDL Particle Number)	579	< 1000	1000-1299	1300-1599	1600-2000	> 2000

Lipids	mg/dL	Optimal	Near or above optimal	Borderline-High	High	Very High
LDL-C (calculated)	52	< 100	100-129	130-159	160-189	≥190

HDL-C	mg/dL 38	**Triglycerides**	mg/dL 57	**Total Cholesterol**	mg/dL 101
	Desirable ≥ 40		Desirable < 150		Desirable < 200

Date Collected	Date Received	Report Date and Time	Requisition Number	Fasting Status
05/14/2010	05/15/2010	05/17/2010 13:11	16014937	NON-FASTING

NMR LipoProfile® test

Reference Range[1]

	nmol/L	Low	Moderate	Borderline-High	High	Very High
		Percentile[1]	20th	50th	80th	95th
LDL-P (LDL Particle Number)	785	< 1000	1000-1299	1300-1599	1600-2000	> 2000

Lipids	mg/dL	Optimal	Near or above optimal	Borderline-High	High	Very High
LDL-C (calculated)	67	< 100	100-129	130-159	160-189	≥190

HDL-C	mg/dL 41	**Triglycerides**	mg/dL 71	**Total Cholesterol**	mg/dL 122
	Desirable ≥ 40		Desirable < 150		Desirable < 200

LDL-C is inaccurate if patient is non-fasting.

Date Collected	Date Received	Report Date and Time	Requisition Number	Fasting Status
05/14/2010	05/15/2010	05/17/2010 13:11	16014937	NON-FASTING

PARTICLE CONCENTRATION AND SIZE

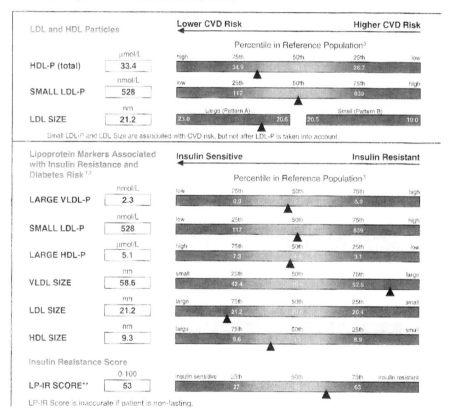

LDL and HDL Particles

Lower CVD Risk — Higher CVD Risk

Percentile in Reference Population[3]

| | µmol/L | high | 75th | 50th | 25th | low |
| HDL-P (total) | 33.4 | | 34.9 | | 26.7 | |

| | nmol/L | low | 25th | 50th | 75th | high |
| SMALL LDL-P | 528 | | 117 | | 839 | |

| | nm | | Large (Pattern A) | 20.6 | 20.5 | Small (Pattern B) | 19.0 |
| LDL SIZE | 21.2 | 23.0 | | | | |

Small LDL-P and LDL Size are associated with CVD risk, but not after LDL-P is taken into account.

Lipoprotein Markers Associated with Insulin Resistance and Diabetes Risk [1,2]

Insulin Sensitive — Insulin Resistant

Percentile in Reference Population[3]

| | nmol/L | low | 25th | 50th | 75th | high |
| LARGE VLDL-P | 2.3 | | 0.9 | | 6.9 | |

| | nmol/L | low | 25th | 50th | 75th | high |
| SMALL LDL-P | 528 | | 117 | | 839 | |

| | µmol/L | high | 75th | 50th | 25th | low |
| LARGE HDL-P | 5.1 | | 7.3 | | 3.1 | |

| | nm | small | 25th | 50th | 75th | large |
| VLDL SIZE | 58.6 | | 42.4 | | 52.5 | |

| | nm | large | 75th | 50th | 25th | small |
| LDL SIZE | 21.2 | | 21.2 | | 20.4 | |

| | nm | large | 75th | 50th | 25th | small |
| HDL SIZE | 9.3 | | 9.6 | | 8.9 | |

Insulin Resistance Score

| | 0-100 | insulin sensitive | 25th | 50th | 75th | insulin resistant |
| LP-IR SCORE** | 53 | | 27 | | 63 | |

LP-IR Score is inaccurate if patient is non-fasting.

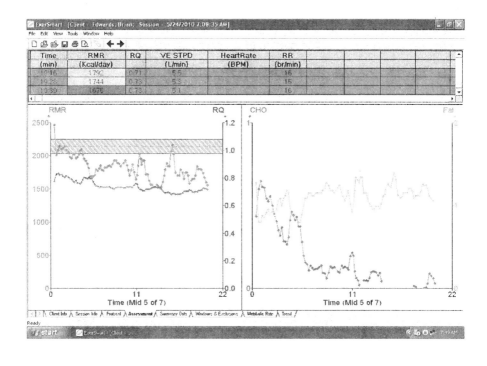

Date Collected	Date Received	Report Date and Time	Requisition Number	Fasting Status
08/28/2010	08/31/2010	09/01/2010 00:13	16290649	FASTING

PARTICLE CONCENTRATION AND SIZE

LDL and HDL Particles

Lower CVD Risk ← → **Higher CVD Risk**

Percentile in Reference Population[3]

		high	75th	50th	25th	low
HDL-P (total)	µmol/L 33.9		34.9		26.7	

		low	25th	50th	75th	high
SMALL LDL-P	nmol/L < 90		117		839	

		Large (Pattern A)			Small (Pattern B)	
LDL SIZE	nm 21.3	23.0	20.6	20.5		19.0

Small LDL-P and LDL Size are associated with CVD risk, but not after LDL-P is taken into account.

Lipoprotein Markers Associated with Insulin Resistance and Diabetes Risk[1,2]

Insulin Sensitive ← → **Insulin Resistant**

Percentile in Reference Population[3]

		low	25th	50th	75th	high
LARGE VLDL-P	nmol/L 2.9		0.9		6.9	

		low	25th	50th	75th	high
SMALL LDL-P	nmol/L < 90		117		839	

		high	75th	50th	25th	low
LARGE HDL-P	µmol/L 7.4		7.3		3.1	

		small	25th	50th	75th	large
VLDL SIZE	nm 62.8		42.4		52.5	

		large	75th	50th	25th	small
LDL SIZE	nm 21.3		21.2		20.4	

		large	75th	50th	25th	small
HDL SIZE	nm 9.4		9.6		8.9	

Insulin Resistance Score

		insulin sensitive	25th	50th	75th	insulin resistant
LP-IR SCORE**	0-100 45		27		63	

Date Collected	Date Received	Report Date and Time	Requisition Number	Fasting Status
08/28/2010	08/31/2010	09/01/2010 00:13	16290649	FASTING

NMR LipoProfile® test

Reference Range[1]

		Percentile[1]	20th		50th	80th		95th
	nmol/L		Low	Moderate	Borderline-High	High		Very High
LDL-P (LDL Particle Number)	651		< 1000	1000-1299	1300-1599	1600-2000		> 2000

Lipids

				Near or above			
	mg/dL		Optimal	optimal	Borderline-High	High	Very High
LDL-C (calculated)	70		< 100	100-129	130-159	160-189	≥ 190

	mg/dL		mg/dL		mg/dL
HDL-C	51	**Triglycerides**	62	**Total Cholesterol**	133
	Desirable ≥ 40		Desirable < 150		Desirable < 200

Patient Name: EDWARDS,BRIAN	Sex: M	Date Collected: 08/29/10
Account: TRADE SHOW VALIDATION	Age: 58	Date Received: 08/31/10
Physician:	DOB: 12/27/1951	Date Reported: 08/31/10
Fasting Status: Not Given	Client No: 00344	Accession: 7424449

The VAP Cholesterol Test

Cumulative Results

VAP Test Results	09/29/09	02/23/10	05/19/10	08/31/10
Total LDL	55	42	95	60
LDL-R (Real LDL)	39	27	86	43
Lp(a)	12	11	4	12
IDL	4	4	5	4
Total HDL	48	40	36	61
HDL$_2$	12	9	4	14
HDL$_3$	37	32	32	48
Total VLDL	14	14	13	17
VLDL$_{1+2}$	5.1	5.2	5.3	7.3
VLDL$_3$	9	9	8	10
Total Cholesterol	117	97	145	138
Triglycerides	58	62	73	70
Non-HDL Cholesterol	68	57	108	77
Apo B$_{100}$	53	48	80	62
Apo AI	140	126	122	170
Apo B$_{100}$/AI ratio	0.38	0.38	0.66	0.36

Other Laboratory Tests	09/29/09	02/23/10	05/19/10	08/31/10

Cholesterol Test

Physician:		DOB: 12/27/1951	Date Reported: 08/31/10
Fasting Status: Not Given		Client No: 00344	Accession: 7424449

Direct-Measured Cholesterol Panel	Actual	Desirable	Risk Low	Risk High	Description
Total LDL	60	<130 mg/dL	▼		LDL-R + Lp(a) + IDL
LDL-R (Real LDL)	43	<100 mg/dL	▼		Total LDL minus Lp(a) and IDL
Lp(a)	(12)	<10 mg/dL		▼	More atherogenic than LDL
IDL	4	<20 mg/dL	▼		More atherogenic than LDL
Total HDL	61	≥ 40 mg/dL	▼		HDL$_2$ + HDL$_3$
HDL$_2$	14	>10 mg/dL	▼		Large Buoyant, more protective
HDL$_3$	48	>30 mg/dL	▼		Small Dense, less protective
Total VLDL	17	<30 mg/dL	▼		VLDL$_{1+2}$ + VLDL$_3$
VLDL$_{1+2}$	7.3	<20 mg/dL	▼		Buoyant VLDL, less risk
VLDL$_3$	10	<10 mg/dL		▼	Dense VLDL, more risk
Total Cholesterol	138	<200 mg/dL	▼		LDL + HDL + VLDL

(handwritten note across HDL rows: "↑ to 1,000 Endurance one")

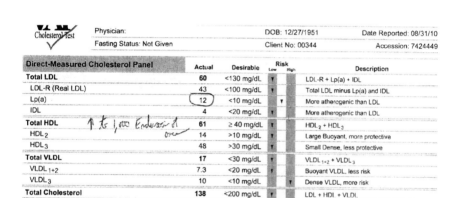

Secondary and Emerging Risk Factors	Actual	Desirable	Risk Low	Risk High	Description
Triglycerides *(AFTER EATING)*	70	<150 mg/dL	▼		Linked to increased risk for CHD
Non-HDL Cholesterol	77	<160 mg/dL	▼		LDL + VLDL
Remnant Lipoproteins	14	<30 mg/dL	▼		IDL + VLDL$_3$
Lp(a)	12	<10 mg/dL		▼	More atherogenic than LDL
LDL Density (Pattern)	(B)	A		▼	B: more risk; A/B intermediate risk; A: less risk
LDL Subclasses (mg/dL) LDL$_4$=16.8, LDL$_3$=23.2, LDL$_2$=3.4, LDL$_1$=0.0					LDL$_{4+3}$ small, dense. LDL$_{2+1}$ large, buoyant

Apolipoproteins	Actual	Desirable	Risk Low	Risk High	Description
Apo B$_{100}$	62	<109 mg/dL	▼		Sum atherogenic lipoprotein particles
Apo AI	170	>118 mg/dL	▼		Sum anti-atherogenic lipoprotein particles
Apo B$_{100}$/AI ratio	0.36	<0.92	▼		Low ratio indicates lower risk

Austin, T)

Patient Name: EDWARDS, BRIAN
Account: NLA- MARCH 2011
Physician:
Fasting Status: Not Given

Sex: M
Age: 59
DOB: 12/27/1951
Client No: 04749

Date Collected: 03/11/11
Date Received: 03/17/11
Date Reported: 03/18/11
Accession: 7878927

Direct-Measured Cholesterol Panel	Actual	Desirable	Risk Low	Risk High	Description
Total LDL	103	<130 mg/dL	▼		LDL $_{4+3+2+1}$ + Lp(a) + IDL
LDL $_{4+3+2+1}$	83	<100 mg/dL	▼		Total LDL minus Lp(a) and IDL
Lp(a)	14	<10 mg/dL		▼	More atherogenic than LDL
IDL	5	<20 mg/dL	▼		More atherogenic than LDL
Total HDL	56	≥ 40 mg/dL	▼		HDL $_2$ + HDL $_3$
HDL $_2$	17	>10 mg/dL	▼		Large Buoyant, more protective
HDL $_3$	39	>30 mg/dL	▼		Small Dense, less protective
Total VLDL	16	<30 mg/dL	▼		VLDL $_{1+2}$ + VLDL $_3$
VLDL $_{1+2}$	7.5	<20 mg/dL	▼		Buoyant VLDL, less risk
VLDL $_3$	9	<10 mg/dL	▼		Dense VLDL, more risk
Total Cholesterol	175	<200 mg/dL	▼		LDL + HDL + VLDL

Secondary and Emerging Risk Factors	Actual	Desirable	Risk Low	Risk High	Description
Triglycerides	78	<150 mg/dL	▼		Linked to increased risk for CHD
Non-HDL Cholesterol	119	<160 mg/dL	▼		LDL + VLDL
Remnant Lipoproteins	14	<30 mg/dL	▼		IDL + VLDL $_3$
Lp(a)	14	<10 mg/dL		▼	More atherogenic than LDL
LDL Density (Pattern)	A	A	▼		B: more risk, A/B intermediate risk; A: less risk

LDL Subclasses (mg/dL) LDL $_4$=7.5, LDL $_3$=38.2, LDL $_2$=31.8, LDL $_1$=5.8

LDL $_{4+3}$ small, dense LDL $_{2+1}$ large, buoyant

Apolipoproteins	Actual	Desirable	Risk Low	Risk High	Description
Apo B $_{100}$	81	<109 mg/dL	▼		Sum atherogenic lipoprotein particles
Apo AI	149	>118 mg/dL	▼		Sum anti-atherogenic lipoprotein particles
Apo B $_{100}$/AI ratio	0.54	<0.92	▼		Low ratio indicates lower risk

5/11
67
163

AUSTIN, Tx (AFTER TRIP TO FLA + LA.)

LIPOSCIENCE

LipoScience, Inc.
2500 Sumner Boulevard
Raleigh, NC 27616
877-547-6837
www.liposcience.com

Page 1 of 1

Patient Name	Sex	Age
EDWARDS, BRIAN S	M	59

Patient ID	Birth Date	Accession Number
16287294	12/27/1951	W0850217

Clinician

SHALAUROVA, IRINA

Client Name and Address

LIPOSCIENCE VIP   20000/
2500 Sumner Blvd

Raleigh, NC 27616
Phone: (919)212-1999   Fax:

Date Collected	Date Received	Report Date and Time	Requisition Number	Fasting Status
03/12/2011	03/16/2011	03/17/2011 06:41	16287294	Not Specified

---

NMR LipoProfile® test

Reference Range[1]

	Percentile[1]	Low	Moderate	Borderline-High	High	Very High
	nmol/L	20th	50th	80th	95th	
LDL-P (LDL Particle Number)	1246	< 1000	1000-1299	1300-1599	1600-2000	> 2000

Lipids

	mg/dL	Optimal	Near or above optimal	Borderline-High	High	Very High
LDL-C (calculated)	110	< 100	100-129	130-159	160-189	≥ 190

HDL-C	**Triglycerides**		**Total Cholesterol**
mg/dL	mg/dL		mg/dL
58	83		185
Desirable ≥ 40	Desirable < 150		Desirable < 200

LDL-C is inaccurate if patient is non-fasting.

NON-HDL-C = 185-55 = (127)

Date Collected	Date Received	Report Date and Time	Requisition Number	Fasting Status
03/12/2011	03/16/2011	03/17/2011 06:41	16287294	Not Specified

PARTICLE CONCENTRATION AND SIZE

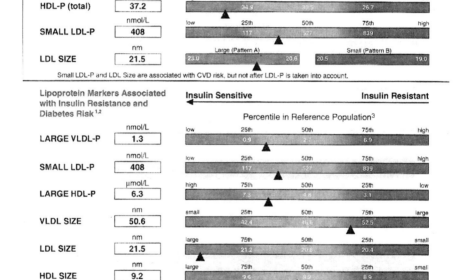

Small LDL-P and LDL Size are associated with CVD risk, but not after LDL-P is taken into account.

Insulin Resistance Score

LP-IR Score is inaccurate if patient is non-fasting

NYC NLA (AFTER 45d cruise)

LIPOSCIENCE

LipoScience, Inc.
2500 Sumner Boulevard
Raleigh, NC 27616
877-547-6837
www.liposcience.com

Patient Name		Sex	Age
EDWARDS, BRIAN S		M	59

Patient ID	Birth Date	Accession Number
15836628	12/27/1951	M0249718

Clinician

SHALAUROVA, IRINA

Client Name and Address

LIPOSCIENCE VIP   20000/
2500 Sumner Blvd

Raleigh, NC 27616
Phone: (919)212-1999   Fax:

Date Collected	Date Received	Report Date and Time	Requisition Number	Fasting Status
05/20/2011	05/23/2011	05/24/2011 09:13	15836628	FASTING

NMR LipoProfile® test

$ApoB_{100}$ 81

Reference Range[1]

	nmol/L	Percentile[1]	20th	50th	80th	95th
		Low	Moderate	Borderline-High	High	Very High
LDL-P (LDL Particle Number)	765	< 1000	1000-1299	1300-1599	1600-2000	> 2000

Lipids

	mg/dL	Optimal	Near or above optimal	Borderline-High	High	Very High
LDL-C (calculated)	55	< 100	100-129	130-159	160-189	≥190

	mg/dL			mg/dL			mg/dL
HDL-C	61	**Triglycerides**	45		**Total Cholesterol**	125	
	Desirable ≥ 40		Desirable < 150			Desirable < 200	

Date Collected	Date Received	Report Date and Time	Requisition Number	Fasting Status
05/20/2011	05/23/2011	05/24/2011 09:13	15836628	FASTING

PARTICLE CONCENTRATION AND SIZE

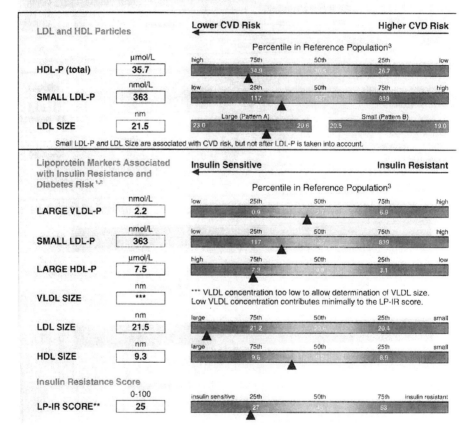

LDL and HDL Particles		Lower CVD Risk			Higher CVD Risk

Small LDL-P and LDL Size are associated with CVD risk, but not after LDL-P is taken into account.

Lipoprotein Markers Associated with Insulin Resistance and Diabetes Risk [1,2]

Insulin Sensitive ← → Insulin Resistant

Percentile in Reference Population [3]

	µmol/L		
HDL-P (total)	35.7		
	nmol/L		
SMALL LDL-P	363		
	nm		
LDL SIZE	21.5		

	nmol/L		
LARGE VLDL-P	2.2		
	nmol/L		
SMALL LDL-P	363		
	µmol/L		
LARGE HDL-P	7.5		
	nm		
VLDL SIZE	***		
	nm		
LDL SIZE	21.5		
	nm		
HDL SIZE	9.3		

*** VLDL concentration too low to allow determination of VLDL size. Low VLDL concentration contributes minimally to the LP-IR score.

Insulin Resistance Score

	0-100		
LP-IR SCORE**	25		

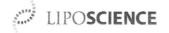

LIPO**SCIENCE**

LipoScience, Inc.
2500 Sumner Boulevard
Raleigh, NC 27616
877-547-6837
www.liposcience.com

Page 1 of 1

Patient Name	Sex	Age	Clinician	
EDWARDS, BRIAN S	M	59		

			Client Name and Address	
Patient ID	Birth Date	Accession Number	LIPOSCIENCE VIP	20000/
16575467	12/27/1951	T0975817	2500 Sumner Blvd Raleigh, NC 27616 Phone: (919)212-1999 Fax:	

Date Collected	Date Received	Report Date and Time	Requisition Number	Fasting Status
08/27/2011	08/30/2011	08/31/2011 10:34	16575467	FASTING

PARTICLE CONCENTRATION AND SIZE

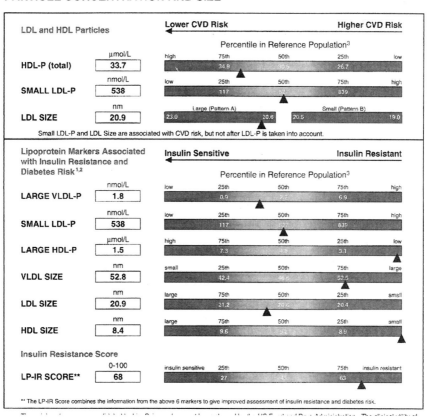

** The LP-IR Score combines the information from the above 6 markers to give improved assessment of insulin resistance and diabetes risk.

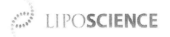

LipoScience, Inc.
2500 Sumner Boulevard
Raleigh, NC 27616
877-547-6837
www.liposcience.com

Page 1 of 1

Clinician

Patient Name		Sex	Age
EDWARDS, BRIAN S		M	59

Client Name and Address

Patient ID	Birth Date	Accession Number
16575467	12/27/1951	T0975817

LIPOSCIENCE VIP   20000/
2500 Sumner Blvd

Raleigh, NC 27616
Phone: (919)212-1999   Fax:

Date Collected	Date Received	Report Date and Time	Requisition Number	Fasting Status
08/27/2011	08/30/2011	08/31/2011 10:34	16575467	FASTING

NMR LipoProfile® test

Reference Range[†]

	nmol/L	Percentile[†]				
			20th	50th	80th	95th
		Low	Moderate	Borderline-High	High	Very High
LDL-P (LDL Particle Number)	1097	< 1000	1000-1299	1300-1599	1600-2000	> 2000

Lipids

	mg/dL	Optimal	Near or above optimal	Borderline-High	High	Very High
LDL-C (calculated)	57	< 100	100-129	130-159	160-189	≥ 190

	mg/dL			mg/dL		mg/dL
HDL-C	44	**Triglycerides**	65	**Total Cholesterol**	114	
	Desirable ≥ 40		Desirable < 150			Desirable < 200

Historical Reporting

LDL-P

400 600 700 800 900 1000 1100 1200 1300 1400 1500 1600 1700 1800 1900 2000 4000 6000

►08/27/11 (1097)

LDL-C

20 40 50 70 80 90 100 110 120 130 140 150 160 170 180 190 200 400

Physician:	DOB: 12/27/1951	Date Reported: 08/30/11
Fasting Status: Not Given	Client No: 02197	Accession: 8303556

Comments

Amended Report

Direct-Measured Cholesterol Panel	Actual	Desirable	Risk Low	Risk High	Description
Total LDL	70	<130 mg/dL	▼		LDL $_{4+3+2+1}$ + Lp(a) + IDL
LDL $_{4+3+2+1}$	52	<100 mg/dL	▼		Total LDL minus Lp(a) and IDL
Lp(a)	11	<10 mg/dL		▼	More atherogenic than LDL
IDL	6	<20 mg/dL	▼		More atherogenic than LDL
Total HDL	47	≥ 40 mg/dL	▼		HDL $_2$ + HDL $_3$
HDL $_2$	9	>10 mg/dL		▼	Large Buoyant, more protective
HDL $_3$	38	>30 mg/dL	▼		Small Dense, less protective
Total VLDL	15	<30 mg/dL	▼		VLDL $_{1+2}$ + VLDL $_3$
VLDL $_{1+2}$	5.9	<20 mg/dL	▼		Buoyant VLDL, less risk
VLDL $_3$	9	<10 mg/dL	▼		Dense VLDL, more risk
Total Cholesterol	132	<200 mg/dL	▼		LDL + HDL + VLDL

Secondary and Emerging Risk Factors	Actual	Desirable	Risk Low	Risk High	Description
Triglycerides	84	<150 mg/dL	▼		Linked to increased risk for CHD
Non-HDL Cholesterol	85	<160 mg/dL	▼		LDL + VLDL
Remnant Lipoproteins	15	<30 mg/dL	▼		IDL + VLDL $_3$
Lp(a)	11	<10 mg/dL		▼	More atherogenic than LDL
LDL Density (Pattern)	A	A	▼		B: more risk; A/B intermediate risk; A: less risk
LDL Subclasses (mg/dL) LDL $_4$=7.6, LDL $_3$=24.2, LDL $_2$=14.4, LDL $_1$=6.1					LDL $_{4+3}$ small, dense. LDL $_{2+1}$ large, buoyant

Apolipoproteins	Actual	Desirable	Risk Low	Risk High	Description
Apo B	63	<109 mg/dL	▼		Sum atherogenic lipoprotein particles
Apo AI	141	>118 mg/dL	▼		Sum anti-atherogenic lipoprotein particles
Apo B/AI ratio	0.45	<0.92	▼		Low ratio indicates lower risk

Patient: Brian S Edwards   **DOB:** 12/27/1951

Lipid Panel: 12/06/2011 09:35

Description	Result	Units	Range	Flags
Cholesterol	145	mg/dL	0-200	
HDL Cholesterol	54	mg/dL	40-90	
Low Density Lipoprotein	76	mg/dL	0-99	
Triglyceride	73	mg/dL	0-149	

LipoScience Lipid Testing: 12/06/2011 09:35

Description	Result	Units	Range	Flags
LipoScience Lipid Testing	16614671	%		

A1C: 12/06/2011 09:35

Description	Result	Units	Range	Flags
A1C	9.7	%	4.0-6.0	H

Comments:
A1C:ᐧ   A1C Interpretive Guidelines:
                         Target value = 6.5%

Estimated GFR: 12/06/2011 09:35

Description	Result	Units	Range	Flags
eGFR-African American	>59	ml/min	>59	
eGFR-Non-African American	>59	ml/min	>59	

Comments:
eGFR-Non-African American: Chronic Kidney Disease is defined as either kidn
GFR less
than 60ml/min that persists for at least 3 months.
    Stage 3 = 30-59 ml/min
    Stage 4 = 15-29 ml/min
    Stage 5 = <15 ml/min
*Patient result is normalized to ml/min/1.73 square meters of body surface
area.

Comprehensive Metabolic Panel: 12/06/2011 09:35

Description	Result	Units	Range	Flags
Sodium	137	mmol/L	136-145	
Potassium	4.5	mmol/L	3.6-4.9	
Chloride	101	mmol/L	99-111	
Carbon Dioxide	29	mmol/L	20-36	
BUN	24	mg/dL	6-20	H
Creatinine	1.2	mg/dL	0.6-1.2	
Glucose	263	mg/dL	74-106	H
Calcium	9.6	mg/dL	8.7-10.5	

LIPOSCIENCE

LipoScience, Inc.
2500 Sumner Boulevard
Raleigh, NC 27616
877-547-6837
www.liposcience.com

Page 1 of 1

Patient Name	Sex	Age
EDWARDS, BRIAN S	M	59

Patient ID	Birth Date	Accession Number
C3201472	12/27/1951	F1102403

Date Collected	Date Received	Report Date and Time	Requisition Number	Fasting Status
12/06/2011	12/09/2011	12/11/2011 23:51	16614671	FASTING

Clinician

SCHEID, JENNIFER

Client Name and Address   15416/

Stormont-Vail Healthcare
1500 SW 10th Ave
Main Campus
Topeka, KS 66604
Phone: (785)354-6692   Fax: (785)354-5072

NMR LipoProfile® test

Reference Range[1]

	nmol/L	Percentile[1] Low < 20th	20th Moderate	50th Borderline-High	80th High	95th Very High
LDL-P (LDL Particle Number)	842	< 1000	1000-1299	1300-1599	1600-2000	> 2000

Lipids

	mg/dL	Optimal	Near or above optimal	Borderline-High	High	Very High
LDL-C (calculated)	67	< 100	100-129	130-159	160-189	≥190

HDL-C (by NMR)	mg/dL 60	**Triglycerides** (by NMR)	mg/dL 48	**Total Cholesterol**	mg/dL 137
	Desirable ≥ 40		Desirable < 150		Desirable < 200

Historical Reporting

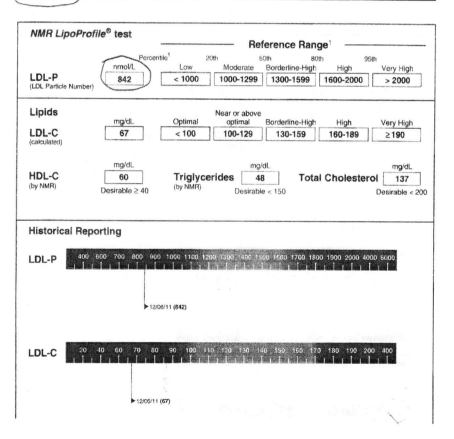

LDL-P

400 600 700 800 900 1000 1100 1200 1300 1400 1500 1600 1700 1800 1900 2000 4000 6000

▶ 12/06/11 (842)

LDL-C

20 40 60 70 80 90 100 110 120 130 140 150 160 170 180 190 200 400

▶ 12/06/11 (67)

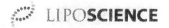
LIPOSCIENCE

LipoScience, Inc.
2500 Sumner Boulevard
Raleigh, NC 27616
877-547-6837
www.liposcience.com

Page 1 of 1

Patient Name		Sex	Age
EDWARDS, BRIAN S		M	59

Patient ID	Birth Date	Accession Number
C3201472	12/27/1951	F1102403

Clinician

SCHEID, JENNIFER

Client Name and Address

Stormont-Vail Healthcare   15416/
1500 SW 10th Ave
Main Campus
Topeka, KS 66604
Phone: (785)354-6692   Fax: (785)354-5072

Date Collected	Date Received	Report Date and Time	Requisition Number	Fasting Status
12/06/2011	12/09/2011	12/11/2011 23:51	16614671	FASTING

PARTICLE CONCENTRATION AND SIZE

LDL and HDL Particles

Lower CVD Risk ◄   ► Higher CVD Risk

Percentile in Reference Population[3]

		high	75th	50th	25th	low
HDL-P (total)	μmol/L 36.0		34.9	30.5	26.7	

		low	25th	50th	75th	high
SMALL LDL-P	nmol/L 289		117	527	839	

		Large (Pattern A)		Small (Pattern B)	
LDL SIZE	nm 21.6	23.0	20.6	20.5	19.0

Small LDL-P and LDL Size are associated with CVD risk, but not after LDL-P is taken into account.

Lipoprotein Markers Associated with Insulin Resistance and Diabetes Risk [1,2]

Insulin Sensitive   Insulin Resistant

Percentile in Reference Population[3]

		low	25th	50th	75th	high
LARGE VLDL-P	nmol/L 0.9		0.9	2.7	6.9	

		low	25th	50th	75th	high
SMALL LDL-P	nmol/L 289		117	527	839	

		high	75th	50th	25th	low
LARGE HDL-P	μmol/L 6.5		7.3	4.8	3.1	

VLDL SIZE	nm ***	*** VLDL concentration too low to allow determination of VLDL size. Low VLDL concentration contributes minimally to the LP-IR score.

		large	75th	50th	25th	small
LDL SIZE	nm 21.6		21.2	20.6	20.4	

		large	75th	50th	25th	small
HDL SIZE	nm 9.4		9.6	9.0	8.9	

Insulin Resistance Score

		insulin sensitive	25th	50th	75th	insulin resistant
LP-IR SCORE**	0-100 16		27	45	63	

** The LP-IR Score combines the information from the above 6 markers to give improved assessment of insulin resistance and diabetes risk.

PATIENT NAME: Brian Edwards
DOB: 12/27/1951
SEX: Male

LAB RESULTS all

12/27/2011 08:15 AM: Ordered/Sent: ORDER:Berkeley Assessment
12/27/2011 08:15 AM: Ordered/Sent: ORDER:Testosterone
12/27/2011 08:15 AM: Signed-Off/Final: ORDER:Lipid*
LIPID*: 12/27/2011 09:27

Description	Result	Range	Units
CHOL	145	107-200	mg/dL
CRF*	3	Men	Women 3.4-5.0
No			
HDL*	45	31-80	mg/dl
LDLC*	86	45-130	
Non HDL Chol	100	LDL + 30	
TRIG	68	35-160	mg/dL

Hemoglobin A1C: 12/27/2011 09:27

Description	Result	Range	Units
HgbA1C	10.0	4.4-6.4	%

08/23/2011 09:45 AM: Signed-Off/Final: ORDER:Hemoglobin A1C
Hemoglobin A1C: 08/23/2011 11:27

Description	Result	Range	Units
HgbA1C	10.1	4.4-6.4	%

960 Atlantic Ave. Ste. 100
Alameda, Ca 94601
(877) 454-7437
CLIA No. 05D0861963

Berkeley HeartLab

LABORATORY REPORT

Report Type	Report Date	Received Date
COMPLETE	12/30/2011	12/28/2011

Requesting Physician

Dr. Scott Towbin
Heart and Family Health Institute

1700 SE Hillmoor Dr. Ste. 200
Port Saint Lucie, FL, 34952

FAX: 7723987974

Patient			
Edwards, Brian	Birth Date 12/27/1951	Gender M	Age 60
ID No. T937511-1	Specimen No. B11175412	Fasting Status 10 hrs p p	Collection Date 12/27/2011

Comments
Pat# 368915

For descriptions of results, see reverse side of this document (or separate sheet)

Arthur Baca M.D., Ph.D., Laboratory Medical Director

		Normal	Inter-mediate	At Risk	Last Visit	Alert Value	ATP III Goal	Reference Range
NCEP ATP III Lipid Tests	Total Cholesterol (mg/dL)	146				>=200	<200	<200
	LDL-C (mg/dL)	79				>=100	<100	<100
	HDL-C (mg/dL)	53					<40	>=40	>=40
	Triglycerides (mg/dL)	70				>=150	<150	<150

		Normal	Inter-mediate	At Risk	Last Visit	Alert Value	BHL Goal†	Reference Range
Advanced Cardiovascular Risk Markers	LDL IIIa+b (%)		19.6			>=20	<=15	13.6 - 43.0
	LDL IVb (%)	2				>=10	<=5	1.7 - 9.8
	HDL 2b (%)		18			<10	>20	7 - 30
	Apo B (mg/dL)		62			>120	<60	<115
	Lp(a), Extended Range (mg/dL)			38		>=30	<30	0 - 30
	Homocysteine (µmol/L)	12.7				>=15.0	<15.0	3.0 - 15.0
	Lp-PLA2 (ng/mL)	162				>223	<200	131 - 376
	CRP (hs) (mg/L)	0.7				>3.0	<1.0	<=3.0
	Insulin (µU/mL)	7				>=25	<25	3 - 25
	NT-proBNP (pg/mL)		419			>450	<=125	5 - 125
	Vitamin D 25 OH (ng/mL)	34				<10	>30	30 - 100

† BHL Goals are intended for patients with established CAD.

Result

Cardiovascular Genetic Marker	ApoE Genotype	3/4
	KIF6 Genotype	Trp/Arg
	LPA-Aspirin Genotype	Ile/Ile

Please refer to additional information for genetic testing results on the Cardiovascular
Genetics Detail Report on subsequent pages.

Test Summary

1 Borderline High LDL IIIa + IIIb with Multiple LDL Peaks, Pattern A region Peak 1 (265 Å), Pattern B region Peak 2 (254 Å)
2 High Extended Range Lp(a)
3 ApoE Genotype: 3/4. See Attached Report
4 KIF6 Genotype: 719 Trp/Arg heterozygous. See Attached Report
5 LPA-Aspirin Genotype: 4399 Ile/Ile homozygous. See Attached Report
6 Vitamin D sufficiency

For Physician Use Only

4myheart Personalized Recommendations

These recommendations have been designed to assist clinicians in developing and implementing a personalized treatment plan for their patient. They are based on the tests in this report and information provided on the BHL Requisition form only. No consideration is made for any previous patient lab values, current diet, lifestyle or drug therapy, or medical conditions. Due to individual patient variability, potential input error, etc., there may be discrepancies between the patient's reported caloric intake value and the appropriate caloric intake value. Clinicians should use appropriate medical judgment in applying these lifestyle therapy suggestions and depart from them in accordance with the patient's individual needs.

Based on the patient height (5' 11"), weight (256 lbs), age (60 yrs), BMI (36) and these Berkeley HeartLab test results, the following is suggested:

* 2400 to 3000 calories from a low (20%) fat diet

* FOOD as POINTS - 46 to 55 points of only "healthy" foods containing:

    CardioProtective POINTS - 28 points

* EXERCISE as POINTS - 11 points of exercise;
  EXERCISE as STEPS - 8000 steps per day

Refer to the education section of 4myheart.com to select handouts for distribution to your patient as appropriate.

The 4myheart Program is available to this patient at no additional charge. Appointments with a Berkeley HeartLab Clinical Educator can be scheduled at 1-800-432-7889, Option 4.

Berkeley HeartLab

960 Atlantic Ave. Ste. 100
Alameda, Ca 94501
(877) 454-7437
CLIA No. 05D0861963

LABORATORY REPORT

Report Type	Report Date	Received Date
COMPLETE	12/30/2011	12/28/2011

Requesting Physician

Dr. Scott Towbin
Heart and Family Health Institute

1700 SE Hillmoor Dr. Ste. 200
Port Saint Lucie, FL, 34952
FAX: 7723987974

Patient		Birth Date	Gender	Age
Edwards, Brian		12/27/1951	M	60

ID No	Specimen No.	Fasting Status	Collection Date
T937511-1	B11175412	10 hrs p.p	12/27/2011

Comments
Pat# 368915

For descriptions of results, see reverse side of this document (or separate sheet)

Arthur Baca M.D., Ph.D., Laboratory Medical Director

Lipid Subclass Detail

LDL-S₃GGE ®

LDL IIIa+b: 19.6%   LDL IVb: 2%

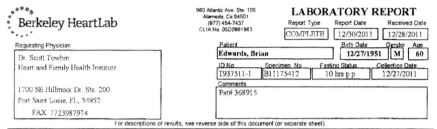

LDL I (%)	19.8
LDL IIa (%)	24.1
DL IIb (%)	31.6
LDL IIIa (%)	16.9
LDL IIIb (%)	2.7
LDL IVa (%)	2.9
LDL IVb (%)	2

	Normal	Inter-mediate	At Risk	Last Visit	Alert Value	BHL Goal	Reference Range
LDL IIIa+b (%)		19.6			>=20	<=15	13.6 - 43.0
LDL IVb (%)	2				>=10	<=5	1.7 - 9.8

Large, Buoyant   Small, Dense

◄── TREATMENT ──◄◄

Atherogenic Subclass Quantitation

	Value	Last Visit	Reference Range
Q-LDL IIIa+b (mg/dL)	13.3		12.0 - 32.1
Q-LDL IVb (mg/dL)	1.7		1.5 - 11.2

	Pattern A Large LDL 263.5 - 285	Pattern I Int. LDL 257.5 - 263.4	Pattern B Small LDL 220 - 257.4
LDL Peak 1 (Å)	265		
LDL Peak 2 (Å)			254

HDL-S₁₀ GGE ®

HDL2b: 18%

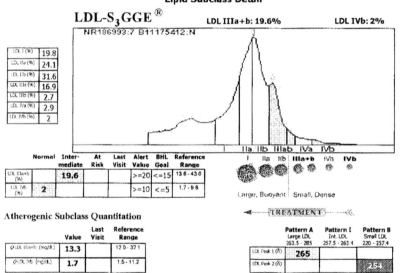

HDL2b (%)	18
HDL2a (%)	27
HDL3a (%)	29
HDL3b (%)	19
HDL3c (%)	7

	Normal	Inter-mediate	At Risk	Last Visit	Alert Value	BHL Goal	Reference Range
HDL2b (%)		18			<10	>20	7 - 30

2b   2a   3a   3b   3c

◄── TREATMENT ──◄◄◄

Healthcare Professionals Only: For help with the use of these test results and recommendations,
call 1 (800) HEART-89 to reach our clinical support line at Ext. 6411

Berkeley HeartLab

960 Atlantic Ave. Ste. 100
Alameda, Ca 94501
(877) 454-7437
CLIA No. 05D0861963

LABORATORY REPORT

Report Type	Report Date	Received Date
COMPLETE	12/30/2011	12/28/2011

Requesting Physician

Dr. Scott Towbin
Heart and Family Health Institute

1700 SE Hillmoor Dr. Ste. 200
Port Saint Lucie, FL, 34952
FAX: 7723987974

Patient	Birth Date	Gender	Age
Edwards, Brian	12/27/1951	M	60

ID No.	Specimen No.	Specimen Type	Collection Date	Time
T937511-1	B11175412	Whole Blood	12/27/2011	8:15am

Comments
Pat# 368915

For descriptions of results, see reverse side of this document (or separate sheet).

Arthur Baca M.D., Ph.D., Laboratory Medical Director

Cardiovascular Genetics Detail Report

TEST PERFORMED	RESULT
ApoE Genotype	3/4

Test Summary

ApoE Genotype: 3/4
* See Guidance Statements

GUIDANCE STATEMENT: ApoE (Apolipoprotein E) Genotype

This patient has the ApoE genotype of E3/E4. The E4 allele can be associated with increased LDL-C levels and therefore an increased risk for coronary heart disease (CHD) compared to individuals with the E3/E3 genotype.

TEST PERFORMED	NONCARRIER	CARRIER
KIF6 Genotype		Trp/Arg
Single Nucleotide Polymorphism = rs20455		(t/c)

Test Summary

KIF6 Genotype: 719 Trp/Arg heterozygous.

* See Guidance Statements

GUIDANCE STATEMENT: KIF6 Genotype

This patient is heterozygous for KIF6 719, with one copy of the KIF6 719Arg allele and one copy of the KIF6 719Trp allele. The 719Arg polymorphism in the kinesin-like protein 6 (KIF6) gene [Human Genome Variation Society nucleotide position NM_145027.4:c.2155T>C] has been associated with increased coronary heart disease (CHD) risk. This polymorphism has also been associated with CHD event reduction from atorvastatin and pravastatin therapy in certain clinical settings. Carriers of the 719Arg allele, either 719 Arg/Arg or 719 Trp/Arg, have a similar increased CHD risk of up to 55% and observed CHD event reduction with atorvastatin and pravastatin therapy in study populations of predominantly Caucasian men and women over 45 years old. Current studies indicate that carriers of the 719Arg allele in an African-American population are at higher risk for CHD and that this risk is likely of similar magnitude to that observed in a Caucasian population. However, the degree of risk and the response to atorvastatin and pravastatin therapy in African-American carriers of 719Arg have not been precisely quantified.

TEST PERFORMED	NONCARRIER	CARRIER
LPA-Aspirin Genotype	Ile/Ile	
Single Nucleotide Polymorphism = rs3798220	(a/a)	

Test Summary

LPA-Aspirin Genotype: 4399 Ile/Ile homozygous.
* See Guidance Statements

GUIDANCE STATEMENT: LPA-Aspirin Genotype

This patient is homozygous for 4399Ile in the LPA gene and does not carry the 4399Met polymorphism. The 4399Ile/Ile genotype is observed in approximately 96% of the BHL patient population. The LPA gene encodes apolipoprotein(a), a component of plasma lipoprotein Lp(a). The 4399Met polymorphism (rs3798220) [Human Genome Variation Society nucleotide position NM_005577.2:c.5673A>G] has been associated with elevated Lp(a) levels and cardiovascular disease (CVD). Position 4399 of the LPA gene is also referred to as position 1891 in public genome databases. In the Women's Health Study, the CVD risk associated with the 4399Met polymorphism was ameliorated by low-dose aspirin therapy. Of note, the CVD risk associated with the 4399Met polymorphism and the amelioration by aspirin therapy has thus far only been observed in a Caucasian population.

SonoCalc™ IMT Scan Report
Common Carotid Artery Intima-Media Thickness (IMT)   V 3.4.0.5

EDWARDS, BRIAN

Date of Birth: 12-27-1951
Age at Exam: 57
Gender: M
Ethnic Origin: White or Other
Patient ID: 9907081
Exam. Date: 12-17-2009
Report Created: 12-17-2009

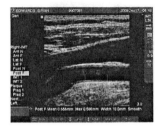

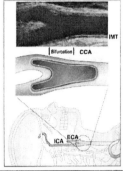

Average CCA Mean IMT:
Average of individual mean IMT measurements

0.599mm

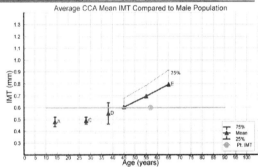

Average CCA Mean IMT Compared to Male Population

Average CCA Max Region IMT:
Average of individual 1mm Max Region measurements

0.741mm

Grossly Unremarkable

12/18/09

Average CCA Max Region IMT Compared to Male Population

A Tonstad, S (1996) Arterioscler Thromb D Tonstad, S (1998) Eur J Clin Invest
B Urbina, E (2002) Am J Cardiol   E Aminbakhsh, A (1999) Clin Invest Med
C Oren, A (2003) Arch Intern Med.

See User Guide for complete references. All reference data is 10mm distal CCA
and is primarily from white populations with no coronary history. Consult your
Doctor for information on race differences.

SonoCalc IMT

Your Doctor should interpret this IMT result in conjunction with your other risk factors. Medical decision making takes a multitude of factors into account, and risk factor modification should be made in consultation with your Doctor.

SonoSite

SonoCalc™ IMT Scan Report

Common Carotid Artery Intima-Media Thickness (IMT)   V 3.4.0.5

EDWARDS, BRIAN

Date of Birth: 12-27-1951
Age at Exam: 59
Gender: M
Ethnic Origin: White or Other
Patient ID: 9907081
Exam. Date: 12-08-2011
Report Created: 12-08-2011

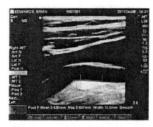

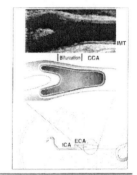

Average CCA Mean IMT:

Average of individual mean IMT measurements

0.563mm

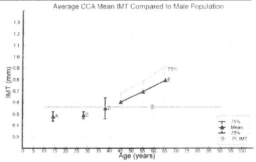

Average CCA Max Region IMT:

Average of individual 1mm Max Region measurements

0.661mm

Grossly Unremarkable

No sign of thickened

Intima/Media or

plaque (>1.5mm).

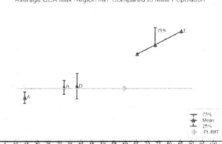

A Tonstad, S (1996) Arterioscler Thromb D Tonstad, S (1998) Eur J Clin Invest
B Urbina, E (2002) Am J Cardiol   E Aminbakhsh, A (1999) Clin Invest Med
C Oren, A (2003) Arch Intern Med.

See User Guide for complete references. All reference data is 10mm distal CCA
and is primarily from white populations with no coronary history. Consult your
Doctor for information on race differences.

SonoCalc IMT

SonoSite

12/9/11

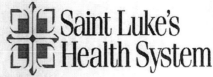

Preliminary Report

Patient name:	**BRIAN EDWARDS**	Study Date:	**12/9/2011**
Patient ID:	**116309**	Height:	**71 inches**
Date of Birth:	**12/27/1951**	Weight:	**200 lbs**
Age:	**59**	Referral:	**Self Referral**
Sex:	**male**	Read By:	
Location:	**PET/CT Plaza**		

INDICATIONS:

Hypertension, Hyperlipidemia, Diabetes

SYMPTOMS:

None

PROTOCOL

High-resolution, ECG-synchronized Computed Tomography (CT) of the heart and coronary arteries was performed using a Multi-Detector Computed Tomography (MDCT) scanner. Each slice acquired was 3 mm thick using a 3 mm slice to slice step. The patient's average heart rate was 105 bpm and varied over a range of 61 bpm. There were no image artifacts..

REPORT

Based on the size and density of the calcium deposits in each artery, a calcium score was computed using Siemens' volumetric cardiac scoring software. Such deposits are markers for underlying coronary atherosclerosis. The coronary artery calcium score enables a person to compare his or her level of coronary calcification to levels found in healthy individuals of the same age and gender. The score is an indicator of the likelihood for significant coronary artery obstruction and the risk of a subsequent cardiac event.

Coronary Artery	# of Lesions	Volume Score (mm³)	Mass Score (mg)	Agatston Score
Left Main	0	0	0	0
LAD	1	3.8	1.23	5.8
LCX	0	0	0	0
RCA	1	2.1	0.81	2.1
Total	2	5.9	2.04	7.9

The Agatston score indicates **Minimal Identifiable Calcification**

Part II

Adjusting to sea change in science.

Tubby Thought

"I (Luis W. Alvarez) remember telling Robert Oppenheimer that we were going to look for {ionization pulses from fission} and he said, "That's impossible" and gave a lot of theoretical reasons why fission couldn't really happen. When I invited him over to look at the oscilloscope later, when we saw the big impulses, I would say that in less than fifteen minutes Robert had decided that this was indeed a real effect and . . . he had decided that some neutrons would probably boil off in the reaction, and that you could make bombs and generate power, all inside of a few minutes . . . It was amazing to see how rapidly his mind worked, and he came to the right conclusions" (Richard Rhodes, *The Making of the Atomic Bomb* [Touchstone, Simon & Schuster, 1986], p. 274).

At the Summer 2010, National Lipid Association meeting in Washington, DC, Penny Kris-Etherton, PhD, RD, CLS, FNLA, at Penn State University, had a change of heart about saturated fats in the diet. She said this when she introduced Dr. Mazafarrian's talk on saturated fats.

At the May 2011, National Lipid Association meeting in NYC, Walter C. Willett, MD, PhD, at Harvard School of Public Health, confessed to the crowd a similar evolution of thought about saturated fats before giving his talk on "Saturated Fat and Carbohydrate: Are They 'One and the Same' Relative to Cardiovascular Risk?"

Chapter 13

Introduction to Part II

I am a diplomate and a fellow of the National Lipidology Association (NLA). I have studied the tapes of the Association of Bariatric Physicians (ABPS), and I am a member of the Obesity Society. The NLA has a bias toward the Mediterranean diet while ABPS has a bias toward low-carbohydrate diets. I hope in this book to bring a balance to the discussion. Present day nutrition is in turmoil. There is little hard scientific data. I will try to concentrate on four studies: A-Z trial, comparative diet trial, and two meta-analysis. These studies taught us the surprising lesson that all the diets are fairly equal in the ability to lose weight and the effect on the lipid profile is neutral. Not what the traditional nutritionists expected. They still tell me that Atkins diet is lipid neutral only if you lose weight. The ABPS says it is not true. I just came back from a forty-five-day cruise and ate all the protein and fat I wanted. I was not hungry. I exercised one to two hours a day. I did not gain weight. My Hgb A1C (diabetes test) improved. This is the main problem with diets. A person can lose weight on any diet. However, after five to ten years, only 5% of people maintain the weight loss. (See Sponge Syndrome.)

I lost 80 lbs. from 2006 to 2007 on the "3-Hour Diet" by Jorge Cruise. I was able to come off insulin. I would meet endocrinologists, and they wanted to kiss me because they finally found a patient who succeeded without bariatric surgery. I could not maintain the 1,500-calorie diet. I hit the plateau and was cold all the time. I was told by NLA that if I exercised 1.5 hours a day, I would maintain my weight loss. After 3.5 years, I slowly gained 50 lbs. despite exercising up to two to three hours a day. My case study is an attempt to bring attention to the cognitive dissonance in nutrition science. As Tom Naughton says in Fat Head, the scientists "have some explaining to do."

I am still in that 5% of successful dieters that have maintained a 10% weight loss after five years. I am still off insulin. I suspect my exercise has helped my insulin resistance the most. My Hgb A1C has started to creep up. I did not want to go back on a 1,850-calorie diet. I had continued to eat every three hours, and I exercised one to two hours a day. I read Gary Taubes's book in January 2011 titled *Why We Get Fat: And What to Do about It.* I also watched his lectures on DVDs from the ABPS. It was an epiphany for me. I have been on a very low-carb diet since January 2011. I no longer eat every three hours. I eat three times a day. I don't get hungry. I also try to eat at least 30 g of protein with each meal. I have not lost weight because I continue to drink alcohol and exercise less. My Hgb A1C has gone down while reducing my Glucophage (metformin) from 2,000 mg to 1,000 mg a day. (Metformin is a diabetic medicine.) Subsequently my Hgb A1C went up off Actos.

ABPS states that very low-carb diets produce a better lipid profile than low-fat diets as it lowers triglycerides and raises HDL. It may raise the LDL-C a little, but the particle size is larger and thus not as atherogenic (not proven). ABPS states that Ornish's very low-fat diet lowers HDL and raises triglycerides. They also say that while LDL-C goes down, the particle size is very small and much more atherogenic (not proven). Atherogenic means "to cause more plaque buildup in the arteries."

Ornish has published data showing regression of plaque with very low-fat diets. He also advises more fish oil if the HDL goes down. However, while fish oil will lower triglycerides, fish oil will raise LDL-C, but it will make larger LDL particles.

Who is right? The NLA or the ABPS?

The authoritative *NEJM* (*New England Journal of Medicine*) has published a trial that shows the lipid panels are the same after two years. However, the authors only report the LDL-C and HDL-C. They do not report LDL-P or the size of the LDL-P. They also do not report HDL-P or HDL size. Thus they do not answer the big question. Also the four different diets look very similar by the end of the two years. The low-carb folks ate more carbs and the low-fat folks ate more fat.

I was shocked to find my LDL-P doubled after six weeks of a very low-carb diet. The size of the LDL-P was large. Were the NLA nutritionists right? Since I did not lose weight, my LDL-P shot up? I was very sedentary while touring in cars. I also drank Guinness. Confounding covariables ruin most nutrition studies.

Whenever you lose weight everything looks better. The problem is, very low-calorie diets lower metabolism and decrease muscle mass. (See Sponge Syndrome.) Part one of my book follows my laboratory numbers as I go on cruises and live the good life on a very low-carb diet while eating more than 2,000 calories a day. No one has documented their advanced lipid tests over the period of a year of dieting.

The first six weeks in January, I drove to Florida. I followed my very low-carb diet quite well except for alcohol. I didn't lose weight, but my Hgb A1C went down. What is amazing is I ate as much as I wanted, and I didn't exercise much, and yet I didn't gain weight.

On the second six weeks I went on a cruise, I ate as much as I wanted, and I exercised a lot. I still didn't lose weight.

Thin folks (Twiggies) from twiggy planet are those that (1) have thin genes, (2) get satiated easily and know they are full, (3) are always moving, and (4) if they gain weight (i.e., from pregnancy) they lose it easily.

Tubbies from plateau planet

1. are prone to apple obesity
2. are more sedentary
3. have metabolic syndrome
4. are prediabetic
5. once they lose weight, they can't maintain weight loss
6. have discordance with LDL-C versus LDL-P. This means that Tubbies often have a fairly normal LDL-C of 120 on their traditional lipid panel. On the advanced lipid test such Liposcience or VAP, their LDL-P or apoB is actually very high and thus have discordance
7. have TG/HDL axis disorder, which means high TG and low HDL and normal LDL-C. This is the dyslipidemia that tubby patients often have. It is part of having the metabolic syndrome.

Tubby Thought

Energy Gap

"According to Hill, a weight loss of 40 lbs. would result in an energy gap of 300-350 kcal. Thus, to maintain weight loss, an individual would have to either permanently reduce their energy intake by an additional 300 to 350 kcal a day or increase their energy expenditure by 300 to 350 kcal per day. This would roughly equate to taking an additional 6,000 steps or 3 miles per day" (Van Dorsten and Lindley, Medical Clinics of North America, September 2011, volume 95, number 5, p. 981).

Caveat emptor:

After losing 8% of your body weight, the exercise metabolic rate decreases by 42%.

Thus the usual formula of burning roughly 100 kcal with each mile of walking is incorrect in the reduced obese.

$100 \times 0.42 = 42$

$100 - 42 = 58$ kcal burned with each mile

Thus a person who has lost all that weight actually has to walk an additional 5-6 miles each day to maintain body weight.

Chapter 14

The Tubby Approach to Diet and Exercise

1. Walk eight minutes after each meal or twenty minutes a day.
2. Cut carbohydrates as much as possible out of your diet.
3. Eat 30 g of any source of protein three meals a day.
4. Don't worry about fats, fatty acids, or cholesterol (trans fatty acid are the exception).
5. Weigh yourself every day. If you are gaining weight, cut back carbohydrates to less than 20 g a day and walk more.

Avoid the "New Year's resolution" advice:

A doctor sees you once a year and tells you to lose weight and exercise. Often, he doesn't specify the diet. He might follow the American Heart Association diet, which is a form of a Mediterranean diet. Fruits and grains should not be the base of a diet. If you are not overweight, it should be at the top of the pyramid. Eat fruit and grains as you would a dessert.

If you are overweight, the experts will tell you to eat 500 calories less a day so you can slowly lose 1 lb. a week. This is an example of giving advice that is impractical. New Year's resolutions fail most of the time. Diets that try to maintain weight loss over five years fail 95% of the time. Something new is needed. Low-carbohydrate diets have been shown to be safe in the A-Z trial and the comparative diets trial.

The worse course is to lose 10% of your weight with a very low-calorie diet such as 1,000-1,500 calories. It will slow your metabolism, and you will gain your weight back in five years even if you exercise two hours a day (my personal experience).

I am advising a low-carb diet (20-80 g a day) as the fat and protein are the best ways to prevent hunger. As long as you are not gaining weight, you will improve your metabolic picture with a low-carb diet as the paradigm that is supreme is carbohydrates drive insulin, which drives fat accumulation and hunger.

We have been misled with the present popular approach:

1. Low-fat diet
2. Very low-calorie diet to lose weight
3. Exercise to lose weight

None of those three items work over the long term. The major source of confusion is which item on the lipid panel counts the most. It is not the LDL-C, HDL-C, or triglycerides or the size of LDL-P. It is all about the LDL-P or the apoB!

If a study or trial does not look at the LDL-P or the apoB, it is meaningless in terms of evaluating the effect of a diet on lipid panel especially in people with metabolic syndrome. People who have apple obesity or the metabolic syndrome usually have discordance of the LDL-P with the LDL-C. This means tubby people will be told they have a normal LDL-C of 120 when in fact the best predictor of heart disease is LDL-P or apoB. Often the number of particles is much more abnormal than the amount of cholesterol (LDL-C). This is discordance.

The bridge between the bias of the NLA and the ASBP and TOS (The Obesity Society) is:

1. find out if there is plaque in the patient with a CIMT and CAC
2. get the LDL-P < 750 with low dose of a statin and Endur-acin.

This is a simple and effective and safe approach. The "New Year's resolution" approach of throwing yourself into a severely low-calorie diet and strenuous exercise will fail 95% of the time over five to ten years. (See Sponge Syndrome.)

Don't try to lose a lot of weight. Control hunger with fat and protein intake. Decrease insulin secretion with low-carbohydrate intake. Check your LDL-P or apoB three times a year. This is very important because there are genetic types who may not do well on a high-fat diet.

Get a CIMT and CAC to determine if you have plaque.

Word of caution: low-carbohydrate diet is very restrictive. However, it is not as restrictive as a 1,500-or 1,000-calorie diet. It is not as dangerous as getting bariatric surgery. It will help a diabetic not go on insulin if you don't gain weight. It will help some diabetics on insulin to go off insulin, especially if you lose weight.

I lost 80 lbs. on Jorge Cruise's three-hour diet. It was great. I ate five times a day. I wasn't as hungry. After a year, I slowly began to gain my weight back, and in retrospect, I think it was the "healthy fruit" I was eating in between meals. I was able to go off insulin, and I am still off insulin despite my 56-lbs. weight gain. I try to exercise one to two hours a day. My Hgb A1C went up from 6.5 to 8.7 over five years. I went on the low-carb diet after reading Gary Taubes's book, *Why We Gain Weight.*

I have been faithful to the very low-carb diet. I try to keep it to 20 g of carb a day. It is four months later. I have not lost weight, but my LDL-P is 750, and my Hgb A1C has gone down to 7.6 while decreasing my metformin from 2,000 mg to 1,000 mg and decreasing my amount of exercise.

I have found it to be a restrictive diet. I miss my weekly bagel. I miss good baguette bread. I miss pasta, but I had already given that up. Since March 2006 (about four years), I tried to avoid the simple carbs such as sugar and white flour products. I tried to get low-glycemic carbs. I didn't eat carbs at night. It didn't matter. Fruit and high-fiber grains in the form of bread or cereal lead to my weight gain. I suffered from the Sponge Syndrome.

The main reason I advise a low-carbohydrate diet is that you can cut down to three meals a day. Eat till you are not hungry and move on. If you get hungry, have a high-protein snack (e.g., cold cuts, hard-boiled egg, kippers). Cook from the Julia Child cookbook and use a lot of butter in your cooking. Every time I am tempted by a wonderful-tasting carbohydrate, I tell myself that if I eat that, I will have to go on insulin. After five months, I find I am not tempted so much by carbs. I think a low-carb diet is easier to maintain than a vegetarian diet.

You don't have to keep a daily diary. You don't have to count calories. You should not eat foods that claim low fat or low cholesterol. Remember, if it doesn't taste good, spit it out.

Tubby Thought

Sponge Syndrome

"A new study published in the *New England Journal of Medicine* finds that hormone changes after weight loss from restrictive diets may make it extra hard to keep the pounds off.

The Study

Researchers at the University of Melbourne in Australia studied the weight loss of 50 obese and overweight subjects over a 10-week period. They found that the changes in hormones that occur during weight loss can last long term. During a deprivation-type diet, hunger hormones leptin and ghrelin, as well as insulin levels change and this study found, a full year after the initial weight loss, hormone levels were still not back to normal. This suggests you may generally feel hungrier than you did months after you reach your goal weight. In addition, you might not be able to clearly detect when you are full, resulting in overeating and weight regain."

Quote from Calorie Count

These are the body's compensatory mechanisms that I call the Sponge Syndrome.

Chapter 15

Weight Loss and Exercise: A False Hope

One: Therapeutic Lifestyle Changes (TLCs)

What are the guidelines?

It is important to simplify the NCEP guidelines. The guidelines advise TLC first. That sets the patient up for failure. There is no diet that will consistently keep weight off for ten years in majority of people. We don't know what we are talking about when it comes to dieting, yet we put the responsibility on the patient to lose weight.

Three items in the news demonstrate our ignorance in weight loss:

1. Jeffrey Gordon: A change in bacteria in the intestine makes it easier to gain weight and more difficult to lose weight.
2. Interleukin Genetics Inc. under the name Inherent Health sells a test for $149 to determine if your patient should be on a low-carb diet or a low-carb-and-low-fat diet.
3. Jerry Heindel is an expert in endocrine disrupting chemicals (EDCs). These chemicals disrupt our weight thermostat. The fat epidemic is not explained totally by video games and corn syrup in fast food.
4. Fetal obesity appears to increase obesity in adults.

It reminds me of how we treated HIV with one drug. Later we realized we did the wrong thing as it allowed resistance to develop in those patients. If NCEP is evidenced based, let's leave diet and exercise out of it for now. We have level 1 scientific evidence as to how to help patients with statins. We should not waste time and resources advising therapeutic lifestyle changes when there are many industries already vying for the patients' attention. There are so many diets because no one diet works. I think we can advise patients to join weight watchers and lose 5% of weight and walk at least eight minutes after each meal. However, this advice should not preclude the diagnosis and treatment of plaque. The patient comes to the physician for prevention of heart disease and stroke. We can do that with statins. We can't do that for certain with diet and exercise.

It is very important to make the NCEP guidelines simple. Taking the TLC advice out of the guidelines will make them simpler.

Two: Diet

Which one is best?

I was giving myself four shots of insulin a day. My friend said if I used all that energy monitoring my glucose with finger sticks and then covering it with insulin shots, why didn't I use that energy to lose weight. I said I like eating too much. But his point was well taken. I could use that energy to write down everything I eat. Unfortunately, only 6,000 people in the National Weight Control Registry have demonstrated that they can maintain this energy or motivation for more than five years.

Three: Exercise, why?

Live longer
Lose weight
Prevent cancer
Feel better
Compete in Senior Olympics

My dad used to say that the best sport is walking down to the bank and making a deposit.

I am reading *Ultimate Fitness* by Gina Kolata. The history of exercise advice from physicians over the years is very interesting. Exercise was popular before the

Depression and then it seemed silly to people. Ken Cooper, George Sheehan, and Jim Fixx helped make it popular again.

In 1960, if you jogged in the street, the police thought you stole something. Fifty years later, I look at my water aerobics class with other old folks and think we have come a long way. The message about losing weight and exercise is already out there. Don't waste three months waiting to see if the patient will do it when a physician prescribes it. I would be upset as a patient to pay for an office visit to be told what I learned in first grade. I have to pay for another visit to start meds? If there was a diet that guaranteed permanent weight loss without staying in a semistarvation state, I would definitely put that at the head of the list of guidelines. There isn't one. We are asking patients to do what is impossible. As for exercise, I learned while studying for the boards that weight loss maintenance requires sixty to ninety minutes of exercise a day. I lost 80 lbs. and exercised 150 minutes a day and still have gained back 50 lbs. As to weight and exercise advice, do we really know what we are talking about? I look at our history of advice and I wonder.

On page 230 of *Ultimate Fitness*, Claude Bouchard is quoted as stating that "weight lifting has virtually no effect on resting metabolism. The reason is that any added muscle is miniscule compared with the total amount of skeletal muscle in the body. And the muscle has very low metabolic rate while at rest, which is most of the time. Skeletal muscle burns about 13 calories per kg of body weight over 24 hours when a person is at rest. A typical man who weighs 70 kg has about 28 kg of skeletal muscle, Bouchard says. His muscles when he is at rest burn about 22% of the calories the body uses. The brain would use about the same number of calories as would the liver. If the man lifts weights and gains 2 kg of muscle his metabolic rate would increase by 24 calories a day. According to Jack Wilmore the average amount of muscle gained after a serious weight-lifting program that lasted 12 weeks was 2 kg. Women of course will gain much less."

The good news is on page 232: "Weight lifting makes for more efficient muscles with more mitochondria and it is better at using fat for fuel. The cells are also more permeable to glucose, which, in turn, reduces the need for excess insulin in the blood. The result is a reduced susceptibility to diabetes."

Will the new guidelines include weight lifting?

I have gone easy on the intensity of exercise and have not had an injury for the last five years. The thirty minutes of hard exercise is doable twice a week, and I started with a trainer about one month ago. I had aches and stiffness all week last week. My trainer said people in her boot camp have been able to get out of their metabolic plateau. Dr. Aronne says exercise is the way to get out of the plateau.

I have not found scientific evidence for this especially when I read that adding 2 kg of muscle only burns 24 calories more a day. In addition, intense exercise burns 10 calories a minute. A 150-lb. man burns 150 in thirty minutes of walking at a 20 min/mile pace. Hitting the metabolic plateau after 7-10% weight loss which decreases metabolism by 42% in exercising muscles dramatically overrides an individual's best attempts to burn calories. I suspect that young people who can do intense interval training for an hour probably are able to overcome the plateau eventually. Once such a person becomes sick or stress prevents him from maintaining such a difficult exercise routine, he will again gain weight rapidly with the Sponge Syndrome. For older folks > 60 years old and even > 35 years old, such intense interval exercise leads to microtrauma and eventual injuries. Exercise is not the way to long term weight loss for the majority of people. Remember also, 10% of people don't respond to exercise.

A person genetically prone to the metabolic syndrome will only maintain his ideal weight by staying in a semistarvation state as per the NWCR data. This mental condition is akin to being a concentration camp detainee as per Ancel Keys data. This is why the philosophy of diet and exercise to lose weight is the psychology of false hope.

Where is the level 1 evidence to decrease mortality with exercise and diet? If there is no level 1 evidence, then it needs to not be the first therapy advised to our patients at risk by the NCEP. If there is no diet that has shown weight loss maintained for more than five years, then the NCEP is advising diet not based on evidence-based medicine. It seems the NCEP should advise only a 5% weight loss and then concentrate on 90-120 minutes of exercise a day for diabetics and prediabetics to increase sensitivity to insulin with emphasis on weight training and cross-training. The new guidelines should also emphasize low-carbohydrate diet for people with the metabolic syndrome. Still, diet and exercise should not be the first therapy.

Four: Fat people lack willpower to change their behaviors?

There is no fat person's eating behavior. Albert J. Stunkark is quoted as saying, "There is no fat person's eating behavior." This defies common sense. Yet Dr. Stunkark has published studies stating this. These studies have been ignored.

The obese are told that if only they would:

1. put their fork down between bits
2. exercise more

3. eat smaller portions
4. count calories
5. avoid fat
6. avoid carbs
7. take the stairs instead of the elevator
8. not eat dessert
9. keep a food diary
10. weigh themselves every day

I have done all the above, and I still gained back 50 lbs. I exercised two to three hours a day. There is no study that shows that doing the above results in permanent weight loss. My question is, why do we continue to preach this? Wittgenstein said, "If you don't know what you are talking about, be silent."

Quoting from *Rethinking Thin* on page 93: "'Most obese people are no different from non-obese people,' Stunkard says. They are not eating because they are depressed or because they have a pathological relationship to food or to their parents. If all you had was their scores on psychological tests–if you could not actually see the people you were testing–you would not be able to decide who was fat and who was not."

http://www.med.upenn.edu/weight/stunkard.shtml

Dr. Albert Stunkard has been quoted as saying, "There is no fat person's eating behavior."

Dr. Stunkard did the twin adoptee studies. Published in *NEJM* 1986, it states, "The adoptees were of the same fatness as their biological parents, and their fatness had no relation to how fat their adoptive parents were."

On p. 122 of the book *Rethinking Thin* by Gina Kolata.

I hope the NCEP takes this into consideration in the new guidelines. We really don't know what is causing the obesity epidemic, and we don't know how to fix it. We do know how to prevent stroke and heart attack with medicine. Simplify guidelines and concentrate on detection of disease and prevention.

Five: Willpower

More from *Rethinking Thin* by Gina Kolata:
Quoting Jeffrey Friedman, p. 144.
"People live in the moment. They lose weight over the short term and say they have exercised willpower . . . It appears that over the long term, this basic drive

(hunger) wins out. And just as willpower cannot make fat people thin, a lack of it does not make thin people fat."

"If your body were as imprecise as you are in counting calories, your weight would fluctuate wildly and unpredictably."

Six: Fat Wars

Rethinking Thin: The New Science of Weight Loss–And the Myths and Realities of Dieting by Gina Kolata.

Important chapter 8: The Fat Wars

Science vs. academics who make a living, promoting diets and others who benefit financially from this moral crisis.

Benjamin Caballero: Eight year, 20 million dollar project sponsored by National Heart, Lung, and Blood Institute followed 1,704 third graders in the Southwest. Despite 27% fat in school diets, increased exercise and nutritional teaching the students did not change their body weight. p. 198. Published in *American Journal of Clinical Nutrition* in 2003.

Archives of Pediatrics and Adolescent Medicine published in 1999 a study of 5,106 third graders for 3 years in California, Louisiana, Michigan and Texas. The control group had the same weights as the group given nutrition classes, more exercise, and healthy food.

David Freedman: People have a wonderful capacity for ignoring negative evidence.

If studies failed to find that changing the environment in schools makes any difference, then the popular solution it seems, is not to question the premise but rather to increase the intensity of the intervention.

When Dr. Pierre-Charles-Alexander Louis found that bloodletting didn't help pneumonia patients, he advised: Bleed earlier and bleed harder.

All the above from pp. 200-201 in *Rethinking Thin.*

The main question discussed in *Rethinking Thin* by Gina Kolata:

How many Americans die each year simply because they are too fat?

See *American Journal of Public Health* by Flegal and Williamson and on April 20, 2005, in JAMA.

Obesity paradox: Since most people die when they are over seventy, having a bit of extra fat appears to be protective, stimulating the body to make more muscle and bone. Williamson says while the paradox is real, the reasons are speculative. The fat wars began in earnest as Williamson and Flegal suffered the exercises of *attack science.*

Fat wars continues

Robert Fogel, Nobel laureate in economics at the University of Chicago found since the Civil war and in other countries that as populations grew healthier, they grew taller and fatter. The best weights for health consistently included ones in the overweight range.

Taken from p. 209: *Rethinking Thin* by Gina Kolata.

Seven:

The science of weight loss is wrong. It is not simply the math of calories in and calories out. The metabolic plateau occurs and the weight loss with the low-calorie diet stops.

Ancel Keys had men of normal weight go on a weight loss diet. Their metabolism slowed by 40%. They became fixated on food. They acted like people from the WWII concentration camps. Jules Hirsch found the obese had numerous and huge fat cells. People who lost 100 lbs. looked like someone who was never fat, but they were different. By every measurement they seemed liked people who were starving. There were a few people in Dr. Hirsch's group that maintained their weight loss by maintaining themselves in a state of semi-starvation. Ethan Sims did a study to get college students to gain weight. He failed. He then used prisoners of normal weight to force them to gain weight. He succeeded. It took four to six months and up to 10,000 calories a day to get them to gain 25 lbs. The prisoners' metabolism increased by 50%. The prisoners' fat cells grew larger but not more in number. After the study, the prisoners had no trouble losing the weight.

References:

Ancel Keys: Metabolism slowed 40% lower than before study started. p. 109. *Rethinking Thin.*

Jules Hirsch: Formally fat people burning as much as 24% fewer calories per square meter of their surface area than the calories used by those who were naturally thin. p. 115. *Rethinking Thin.*

Ethan Sims: When thin men got fat, their metabolism increased by 50%. p. 118. *Rethinking Thin.*

Michael Rosenbaum and Rudolph Leibel found that people who lost about 10% of their weight, reduced the amount of calories burned during movement by 42%. p. 113, *The Skinny: On Losing Weight.*

My diet history:

February 2006: 280 lbs. and taking insulin four to five times a day.

June 2007: 200 lbs., 1,500 calories a day. I couldn't lose any more weight. I was cold all the time. I exercised two hours a day.

I decided to eat more and build my muscle to try to get out of the metabolic plateau.

How many calories and how much exercise should I do?

200 lbs., basal metabolic rate.
$200 \times 10 = 2,000$ calories (I later learned that the NWCR advises 7 cal/lb.)

Two hours moderate exercise: 800 calories.
(A 150-lb man burns 150 calories with thirty minutes brisk walking; hence, I calculate that a 200-lb man burns 400 calories with moderate exercise over one hour.)

I increased my diet to 2,800 calories a day and ate every three hours. I increased the protein and avoided carbs and desserts.

May 2010: 250 lbs.

I have a personal trainer. I did water aerobics because I was worried that my usual treadmill walking and weight lifting circuit on the weight machines decreased my calorie burning due to muscle memory.

I regained a lot of the muscle I had lost during the dieting. I thought I could improve my metabolism. The NLA teaches that weight maintenance can be achieved with ninety minutes of exercise a day.

Then I read *Ultimate Fitness* by Gina Kolata. On page 230, Claude Bouchard states, "Weight lifting has virtually no effect on resting metabolism . . . Skeletal muscle burns about 13 calories per kg. of body weight over 24 hours when a person is at rest . . . If a man lifts weights and gains 2 kg. of muscle his metabolic rate would increase by 24 calories a day."

Back to the question: how many calories should I have eaten to maintain my 200 lbs.?

Basal metabolism reduced by 40% due to metabolic plateau = 1,200 calories.

Exercise metabolism reduced by 40% also = $800 \times 0.4 = 800 - 320 = 480$ calories.

Thus to maintain my weight of 200 lbs. with two hours of moderate exercise, I had to stay on 1,680 calories a day for the rest of my life. (I later learned the NWCR would have me eat 1,400 calories a day and walk 5 miles a day to maintain my weight of 200 lbs.)

Does anyone wonder why diets don't work? It is not a matter of willpower or changing behavior.

Apparently, metabolism decreases by 2% every decade after age thirty. At age sixty, my metabolism has decreased by 6%.

1,200 calories $\times$ 0.06 = 72 calories.

So now I am down to 1,610 calories a day. If I did the same routine of exercise each day, I would lose 10%.
480 calories $\times$ 0.10 = 48 calories.

Now I am down to 1,560 calories a day with two hours of moderate exercise just to maintain my weight of 200 lbs. This is a life of semistarvation. There are very few people who have done this for over ten years or more. Can we please leave the TLC (therapeutic life style changes) off the NCEP guidelines if we can't tell people how to keep the weight off.

Tubby Thought

The Sponge Syndrome Protects Humans from Starvation

"THE PHYSIOLOGICAL SYSTEM CONTROLLING FOOD INTAKE AND ENERGY EXPENDITURE ...

One common misconception is that this physiological system is dedicated to the prevention of obesity. Instead this system's essential role is in the prevention of starvation (i.e., ensuring adequate energy intake to compensate for the energy requirements of basal metabolism, physical activity, growth, and reproduction). As a result, this physiological system is more strongly biased toward prevention of energy deficiency rather than excess storage."

From Greenspan's endocrine text

Chapter 16

Obesity Core Conference 10-1-2011

Exercise with Tim Church:

Dr. Church presented his findings from a study he did with RT vs. Aerobic vs. RT + Aerobic. All exercised the same total amount. All ate the same amount of calories.

The RT (resistance training) group kept getting stronger but didn't lose weight.

The RT (weight lifting) + aerobic lost the most weight.

People liked the RT exercise but found the aerobic exercise boring.

He also cited the data for exercise preventing heart disease.

Ten minutes a day has the greatest benefit to prevent heart disease.
Thirty minutes is a little better.
More than that improves outcomes very little in relation to the amount of work required.
If you are a 10 km runner, you don't improve your outcomes by being a marathon runner.

Three years ago the federal government made guidelines for exercise.

www.health.gov/paguidelines

Achieving Target Levels of Physical Activity: The Possibilities Are Endless

These examples show how it's possible to meet the guidelines by doing moderate-intensity or vigorous-intensity activity or a combination of both. Physical activity at this level provides substantial health benefits.

Ways to get the equivalent of 150 minutes (2 hours and 30 minutes) of moderate-intensity aerobic physical activity a week plus muscle-strengthening activities:

- Thirty minutes of brisk walking (moderate intensity) on 5 days, exercising with resistance bands (muscle strengthening) on 2 days;
- Twenty-five minutes of running (vigorous intensity) on 3 days, lifting weights on 2 days (muscle strengthening);
- Thirty minutes of brisk walking on 2 days, 60 minutes (1 hour) of social dancing (moderate intensity) on 1 evening, 30 minutes of mowing the lawn (moderate intensity) on 1 afternoon, heavy gardening (muscle strengthening) on 2 days;
- Thirty minutes of an aerobic dance class on 1 morning (vigorous intensity), 30 minutes of running on 1 day (vigorous intensity), 30 minutes of brisk walking on 1 day (moderate intensity), calisthenics (such as sit-ups, push-ups) on 3 days (muscle strengthening);
- Thirty minutes of biking to and from work on 3 days (moderate intensity), playing softball for 60 minutes on 1 day (moderate intensity), using weight machines on 2 days (muscle-strengthening on 2 days); and
- Forty-five minutes of doubles tennis on 2 days (moderate intensity), lifting weights after work on 1 day (muscle strengthening), hiking vigorously for 30 minutes, and rock climbing (muscle strengthening) on 1 day.

Ways to be even more active

For adults who are already doing at least 150 minutes of moderate-intensity physical activity, here are a few ways to do even more. Physical activity at this level has even greater health benefits.

- Forty-five minutes of brisk walking every day, exercising with resistance bands on 2 or 3 days;
- Forty-five minutes of running on 3 or 4 days, circuit weight training in a gym on 2 or 3 days;

- Thirty minutes of running on 2 days, 45 minutes of brisk walking on 1 day, 45 minutes of an aerobics and weights class on 1 day, 90 minutes (1 hour and 30 minutes) of social dancing on 1 evening, 30 minutes of mowing the lawn, plus some heavy garden work on 1 day;
- Ninety minutes of playing soccer on 1 day, brisk walking for 15 minutes on 3 days, lifting weights on 2 days; and
- Forty-five minutes of stationary bicycling on 2 days, 60 minutes of basketball on 2 days, calisthenics on 3 days.

Tim Church's Ultimate Workout:
High intensity one day a week
Resistance training 1-2 d a week
Aerobic 45-60 minute a day
Stretching 4-5 days a week

Blair, JAMA 1989, 262:2395
30 minutes of walking five days a week

DREW study Church et al.
HART-D
JAMA Nov 2010

Behavioral Therapy by Suzanne Phelan, PhD

Dr. Phelan said they have the most research with the best results? But they cherry pick their patients.

1950s Freud said it was all about oral fixation

1967 Stuart had his patient seen seven times a week and weighed themselves four times a day
He practiced cognitive therapy and positive reinforcement. He had a 16-kg weight loss in eight patients.

1970s Group Therapy was tried.

Tools to Modify Behavior:
Record food intake and feelings
Record weight and activity
Record immediately
Encourage honesty

Review weekly with patient
Goal setting
Rewards
Response to SLIPS in the program.
Cognitive restructuring (like sad to glad)
Modify maladaptive thought patterns

Reference:

Wadden Obes Res2004
Attrition 21.2% over thirty-six months.
Tsai, Wadden, 2009, J. Gen Int Med, 24(9). Very important reference
Galuska JAMA 1999 having the doctor say something helps

No behavioral predictors as to who will do well with behavioral treatment.

Behavioral Treatment:
Done at Academic Research Center
Free Rx.
Intensive Rx.
Patients are screened.
One hour meeting once a week for the first six months
Biweekly meetings thereafter.

Perri, JCCP 1988; 56, pp. 529-534.

Learn behaviors–unlearn or modify behaviors–by changing the environment.

This was very interesting. They cherry pick their patients. They spend a tremendous amount of time with them. The patients are very dedicated. They still have a large drop out?

This program is not practical for a large group.

I asked her Dr. Phelan about the Midtown Manhattan Study in 1965 with Mickey Stunkard not finding a behavior that obese have which thin people do not have. She was a student of Mickey's but she did not know what I was talking about.

Chris Gardner: A-Z trial

Recent trials before 2009 were small and short duration. The best trial after 2009 is Sachs's comparative diet trial. However, Chris says by the end of the Sachs trial, the four diets are not very different from each other.

2008 trial was good: Shai 2008, *NEJM*, 359, p. 359, Low Fat vs. Low Carb. (low carb won)

The A-Z trial had four diets. All ate the same amount of calories despite eat all you want on Atkins and Ornish.

The Waterfall slide shows every patient in the trial as to how much weight they gained or lost. Within groups there is a 30 lb. difference in weight loss to weight gain.

Atkins and Ornish easier to follow as you eat foods without carbs or without fats.

By the end of the trial they were significantly different. Ornish 15% fat. Atkins 22% carb with more protein.

High protein diets always win because of satiety. Which type of protein? What is the long term effect of protein on liver and kidney that have to remove the nitrogen as ammonia?

Chris says that there will be no more head to head macronutrient diets.

It will be tailored diets based on insulin resistance and genetics. People with CC genotype do better on low fat.

References from Chris:

McLaughlin: Arch Internal Medicine 2007, 167, p. 642
Cornier obesity research 205, 13(4), p. 703-9
Pittas
Qi et al., Circulation 2011, 124, p. 565-571

Chris says people can tolerate 20% carb. Most patients prefer 40%.

Pearls from other speakers:
Frank Greenway said the ADA (American Diabetic Association) advised:

Carb 40%

Fat 40%

Protein 20%

The epidemiologists got the ADA to change to low-fat diet.
The Mediterranean diet usually allows up to 55% fat.

Frank Greenway: You will lose the excess fat cells after a few years at low maintenance weight

Dan Bessensen: Once you diet you become more energy efficient. It might take two years for it to go up.

Once you lose weight you reach plateau when you reach low leptin level.

The fat cells produce the leptin. As they shrink they produce less leptin.
Once the leptin gets low you get hungry and your metabolism slows down.

Dan also said Lap Band requires frequent follow up by the surgeon to adjust the lap band.

Dan said the Roux en Y bypass has a 50% decrease in fat excess. He said this means 25% loss of total body weight. So after five years this surgery has maintained a 25% total body weight loss. There are 20% that fall out of the program. Jim believes they are over-estimating the long term success of bariatric surgery.

It doesn't matter how you lose weight. The problem is how to maintain weight. Dr. Jim said he just published something about the Hawaiians doing well because of a spiritual community. He had a 21% drop out rate. Jim doesn't put much stock in the behavioral treatment.

National Weight Control Registry

This section presented a woman on weight watchers who hit plateau or settlement point. What should be done next? I said Dr. Aronne wrote in his book that she should not decrease her calories more. The facilitator suggested that the 240 calorie gap be made up by exercise and diet. I said that is virtually impossible. Dr. Aronne writes that after 8% body weight loss the patients exercise metabolism goes down by 42%. This means that the patient will not burn 100 calories after walking a mile. She will only burn 60 calories. I could believe that walking another 2.5 miles a day is possible but not another 4 miles a day. The facilitators said the people in the NWCR scored high on the cognitive restraint subscale.

This group of extraordinary people did the following:

1.   weigh themselves every day and then if 3-5 lbs. heavier, they had a plan what to do about it immediately
2.   they tended to have little variety in their food
3.   they splurged less on food on holidays.
4.   they ate 1,385 calories/day but the facilitator said they are under reporting
5.   they ate 4.87 meals a day
6.   they linked behaviors to something more than just losing weight. For example they use walking as their social time. They linked good behaviors to something they want to do.
7.   they often had a life changing advent such as divorce or new job.

I went from 280 to 200 pounds and then hit the plateau or new settlement point. I had been eating 1400 calories a day and could not lose weight. I thought that if I wanted to maintain weight I should eat 10 calories per pound or 2,000 calories. I gained back 58 lbs. over four years despite two to three hours of exercise a day. The facilitator said they advise 7 calories per pound.

I said, look at me, do you think I can live on 1,400 calories a day and walk 5 miles a day?

This was the nail in the coffin for low-calorie diets for me. These low-calorie diets take you to a place in your physiology that only 5% of the population can sustain.

Dr. Louis Aronne: Drugs for Obesity

He gave an off-label indication for phentermine. It is used only for six months to curb appetite. He has many people take it chronically. He has the patient sign a consent form. He usually only has to give 18.5 mg, which is one-half tablet a day.

In his book, *The Skinny On Losing Weight Without Being Hungry*, he lists many medications that may cause the patient to gain weight. Actos can cause weight gain in Diabetes. Dr. Aronne would switch his patients to Victoza to avoid that side effect. The generic name is Liraglutide and is given 3.0 mg injectable once a day.

The last four drugs brought before the FDA board were turned down. There seems to be a bias against obesity drugs, perhaps a feeling that people simply need more discipline, similar to the Chris Christie silliness when it was said he didn't have enough discipline to be president as evidenced by his weight. Dr. Aronne told a student of his, who had a similar attitude toward the obese, not to eat anything for twenty-four hours other than water. The next morning he told Dr. Aronne that he had to eat something around 3:00 AM.

Viagra is known to cause a rare case of blindness. It is still on the market. People died taking Viagra and nitroglycerin. No one died from valve disease from phentermine in the Phen-fen treatment. A few people did have their valves replaced. This was a combination that worked very well. The FDA should have just put a black box warning on it and required lower doses. The black box should require physicians to do a screening echocardiograms and follow-ups in a year. Instead, we are doing Roux en Y gastric bypass surgeries with mortalities as high a one in 200 surgeries. Now that we have obesity crisis, Dr. Aronne believes the FDA will ease up on criteria for accepting obesity drugs.

Orlistat works well with some people. It prevents absorption of fat. I was on it and discovered after a fart on the bed that the oily secretion went through my underpants, pants, bed cover, and two sheets to the mattress. Xenical (Orlistat) is over the counter at a lower dose as Alli 60 mg.

Dr. Aronne suggests taking Orlistat for constipation that occurs as a result of dieting.

Dr. Aronne says that the body uses several compensatory mechanisms to prevent weight loss. This is why the future will be combination therapy to treat obesity. Leptin has been given with another drug only to result in antibodies against the leptin.

Combination therapy has made treating hypertension, diabetes mellitus type II, HIV, and hyperlipidemia safer and more effective.

Dr. Aronne said he tried to get his hospital to let him do a trial with B-HCG. They refused on the basis it had been done already with ten trials in the seventies. Those studies determined B-HCG was only a placebo effect. Shetty, KR Arch Intern Med1977.

Dr. Aronne said Zantrex-3 has four different types of caffeine in it. This and other over the counter treatments for obesity have not been proven to help weight loss.

Bariatric Surgery: Chris Still, MD

Dr. Still says this is the only long term safe and effective treatment modality for metabolic abnormalities of obesity. He advises sending patients to a Center of Excellence. His mortality rate is 0.15. I had heard it was one in 200 on the *Today* show when Al had his bariatric surgery. Dr. Still said thromboembolism was the most common cause of death.

Outcome: 20% gain back weight.

There is 50% loss of excess weight. I was told to consider this means 25% of total weight. People with a bad genotype often don't lose much weight.

Future of Treating Obesity: David Allison, PhD
School exercise doesn't work. CMJ 2009, 180(7): 719-26

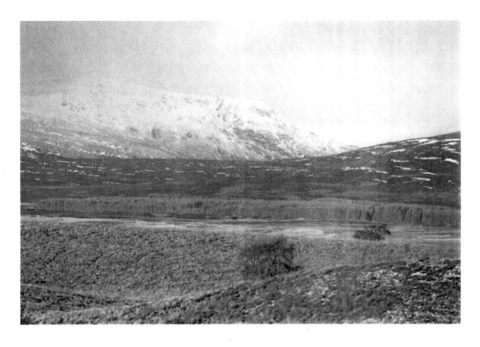

Scotland

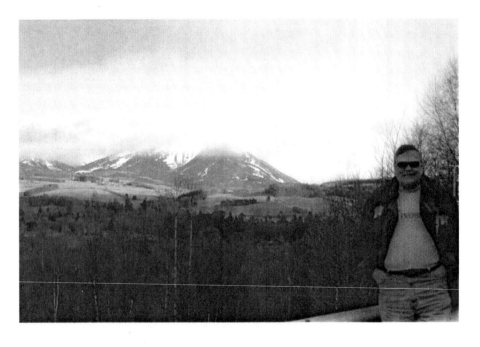

Scotland with Brian

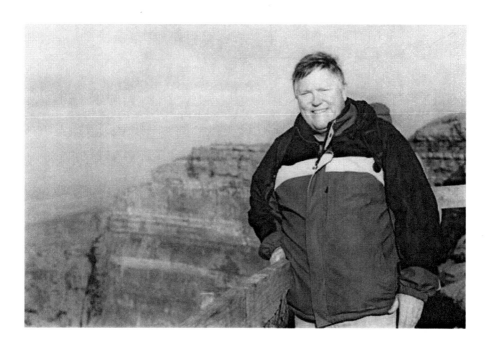

Cliffs of Moher, Ireland

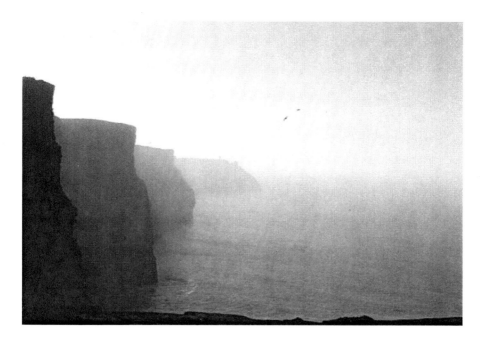

Cliffs of Moher, Ireland

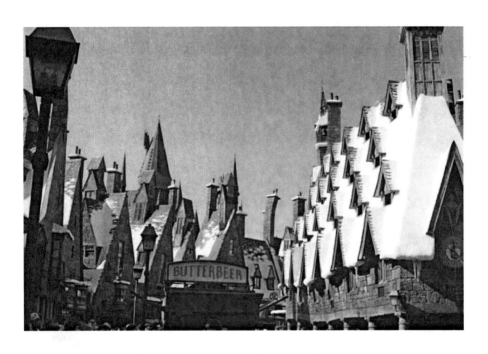

Harry Potter at Universal Studios in Orlando

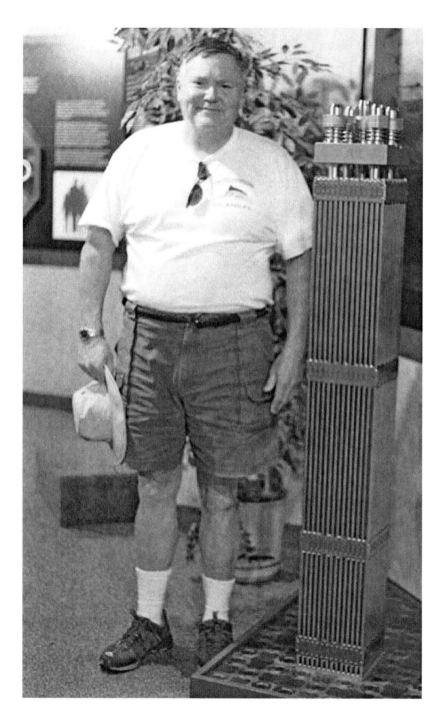

Fuel Rods at Nuclear Power plant in Florida

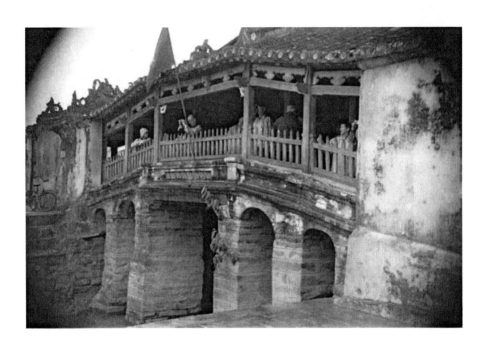

Japanese bridge in Viet Nam

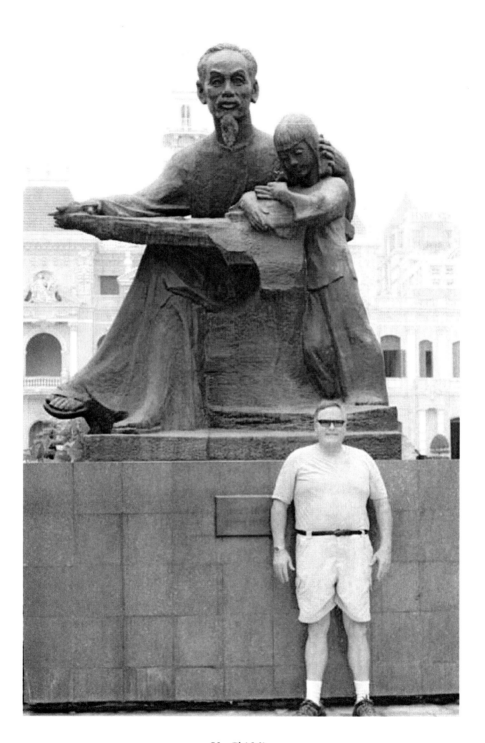

Ho Chi Min

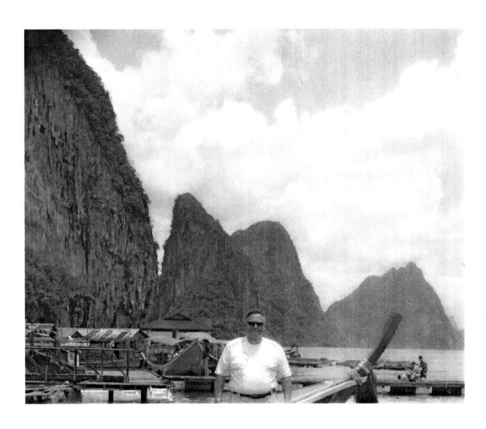

Phuket, Thailand

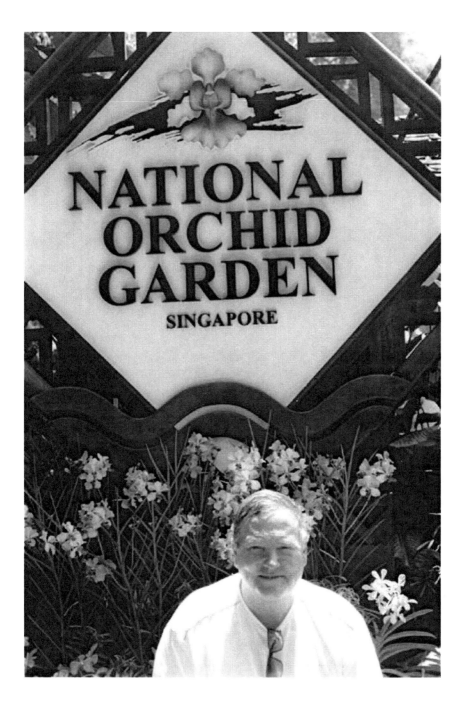

Singapore

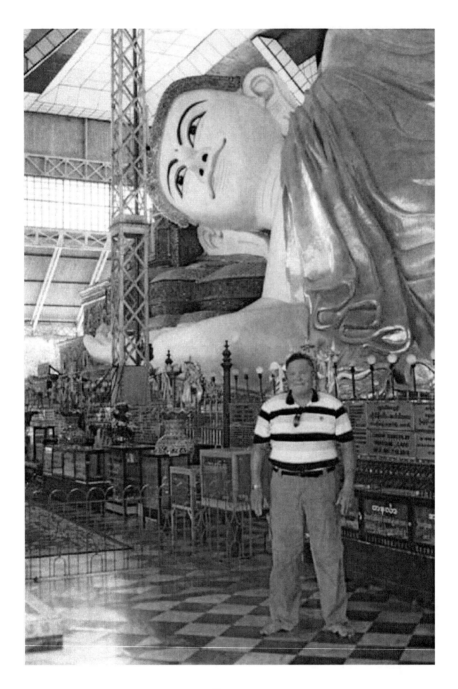

Burma

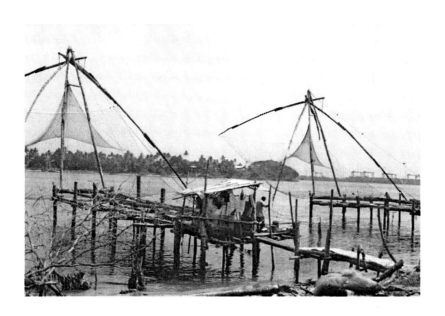

Chinese Fishing Nets in India

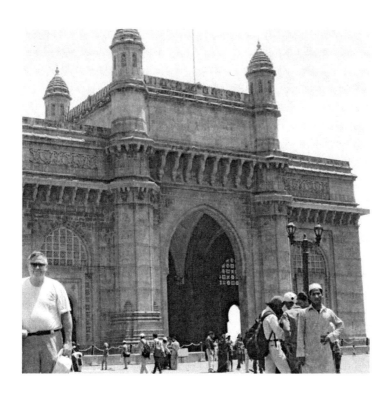

Gateway to India

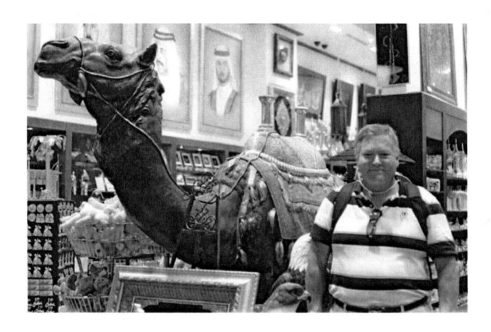

Mumbai Mall

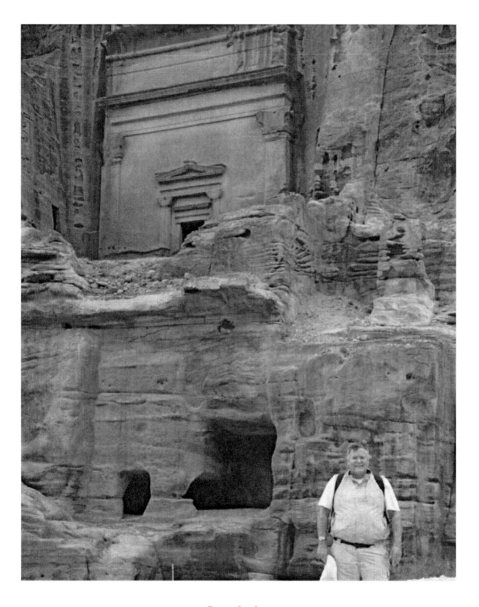

Petra, Jordan

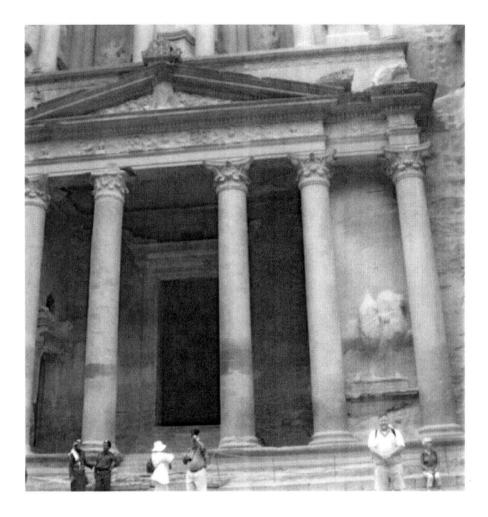

Petra

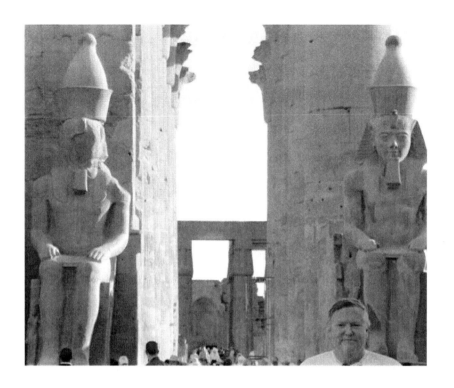

Luxor, Egypt

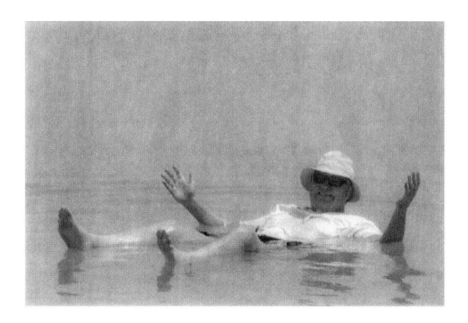

Dead Sea

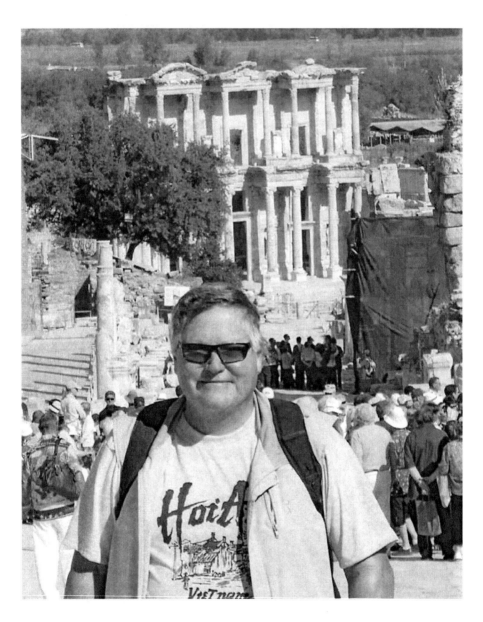

Ephesus, Turkey

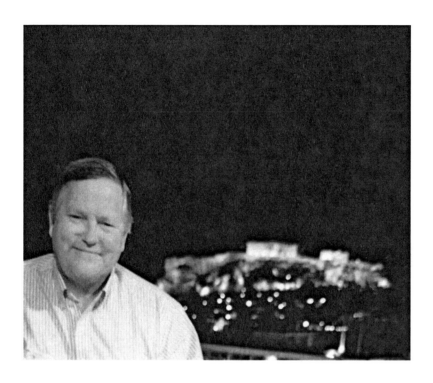

Acropolis, Athens

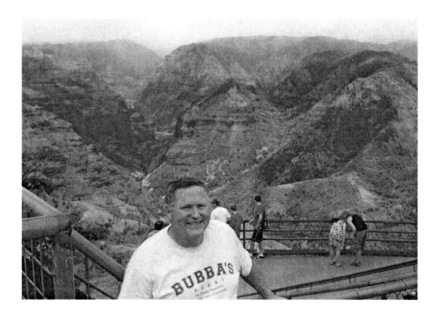

Waimea, Hawaii

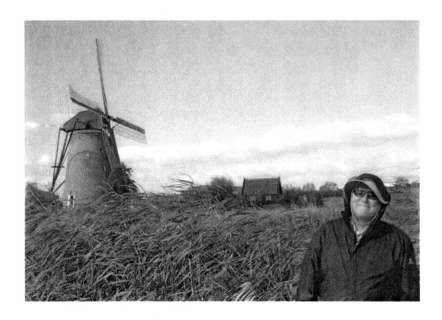

Holland

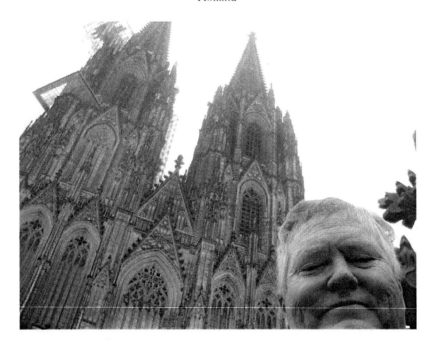

Cologne Cathedral. After it was built it was the tallest structure in Europe
until France built the Eiffel Tower.

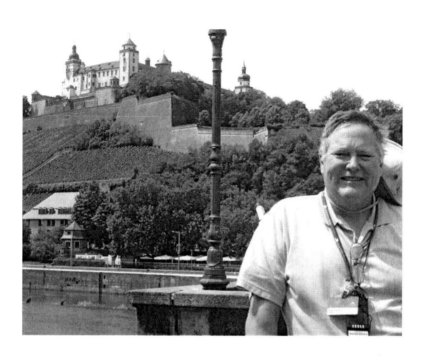

Rhine castle

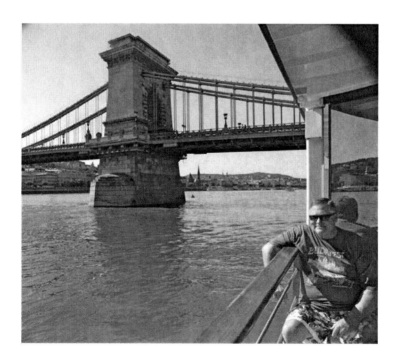

Budapest

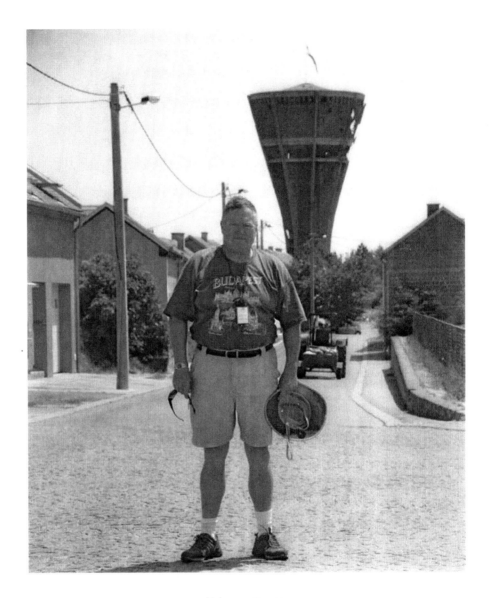

Vukovar, Croatia

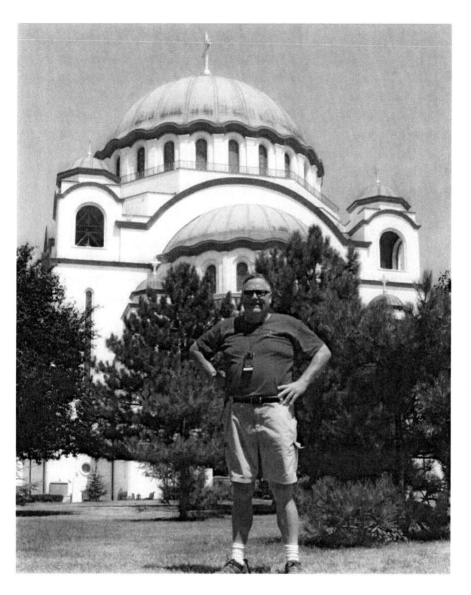

Belgrade, Serbia

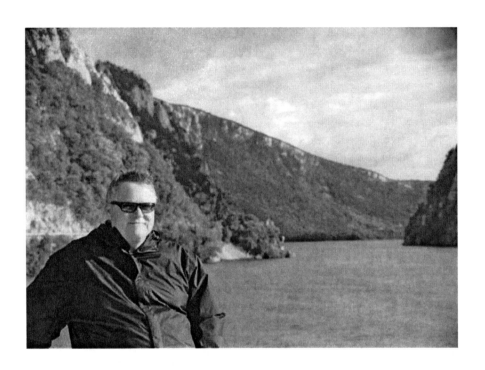

On the Danube

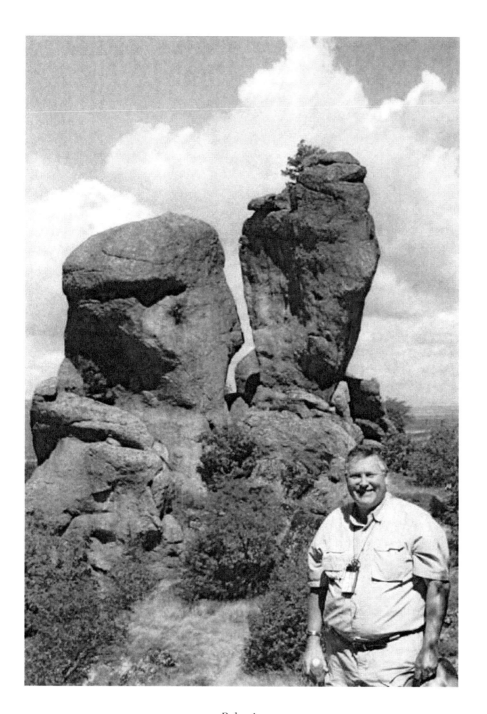

Bulgaria

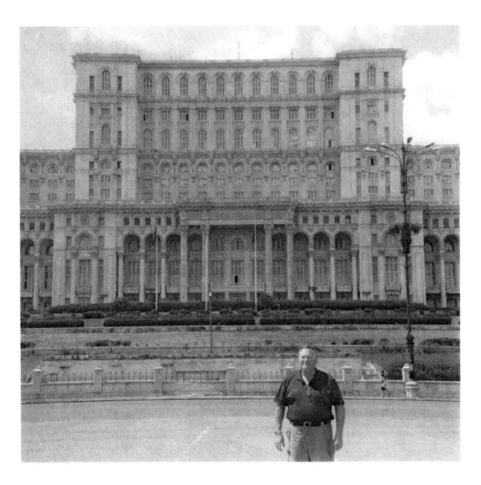

Bucharest Parliament Building

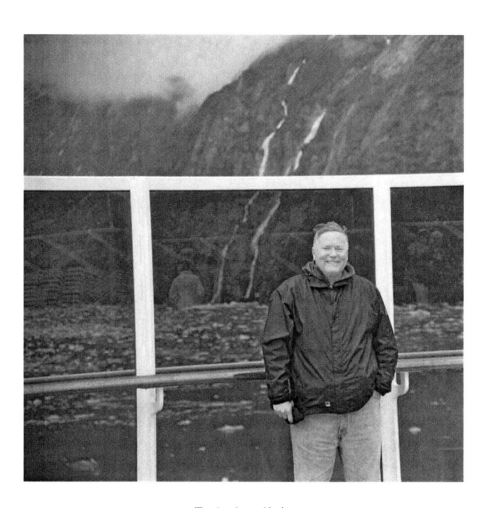

Tracies Arm, Alaska

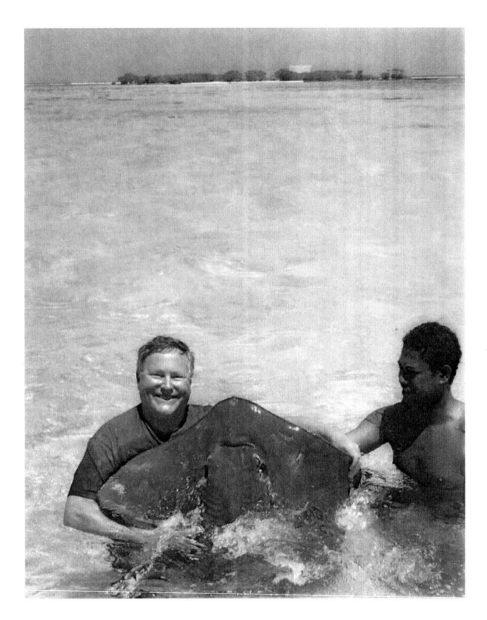

Bora Bora Mantra Ray

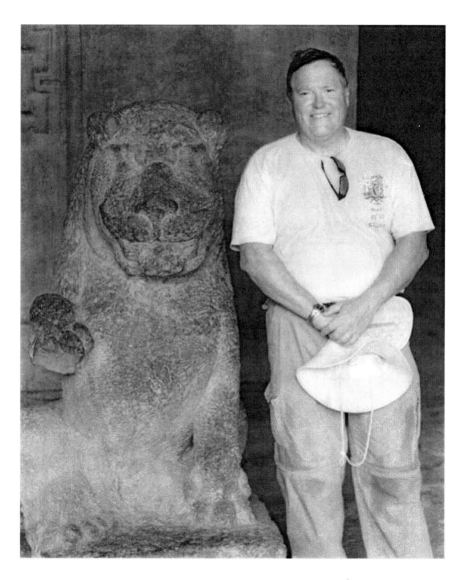

Elephanta, India

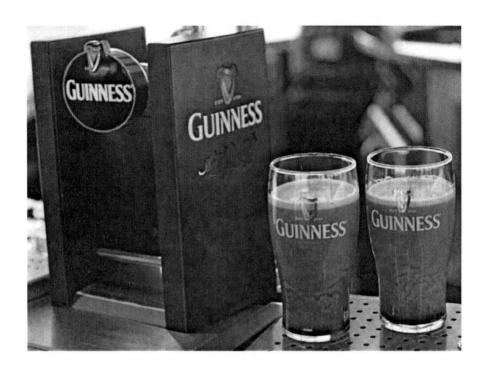

A Proper pour of Guinness Beer

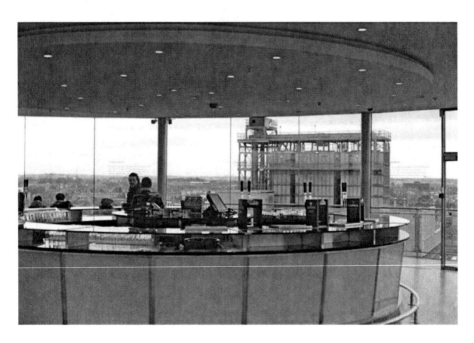

Guinness Observatory Tower–Best view in Dublin

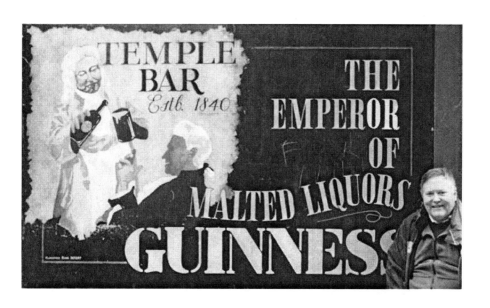

Temple bar

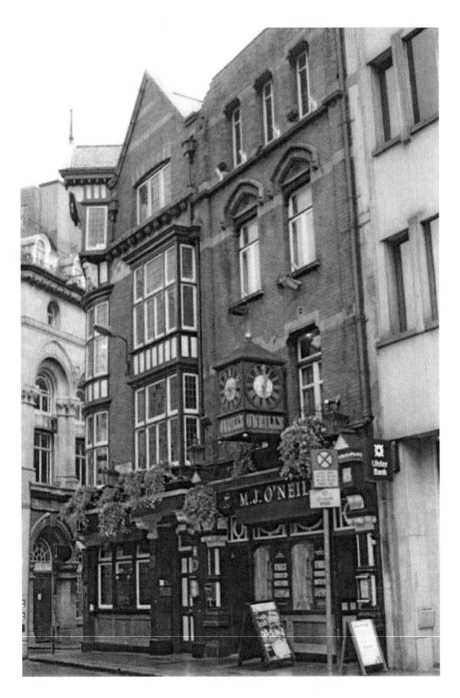

O'Neil's Pub in Dublin—great place for lunch or dinner

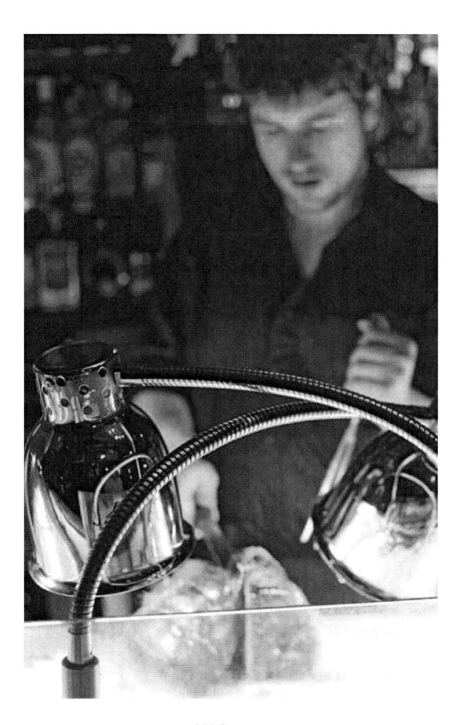

O'Neil's carvary

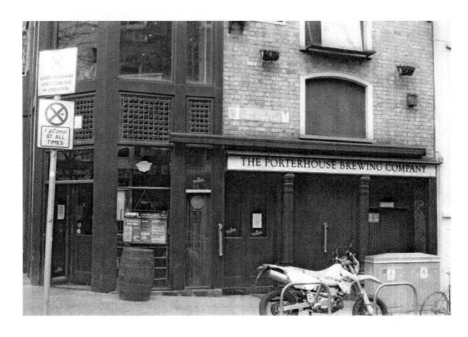

Porterhouse Brewing Company—My favorite pub in the Temple Bar area in Dublin

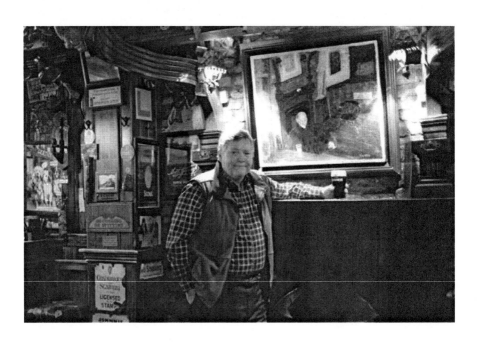

My favorite pub is Gertie Brown's

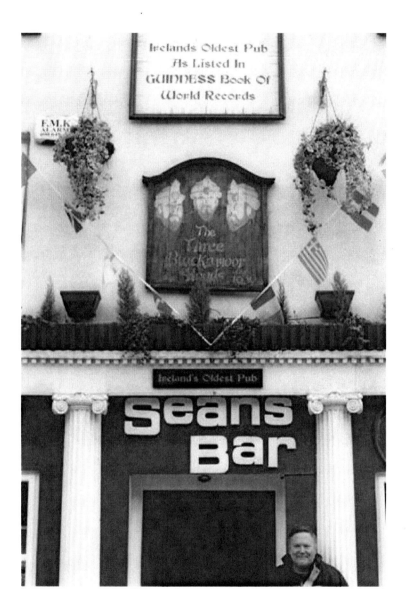

Ireland's oldest pub

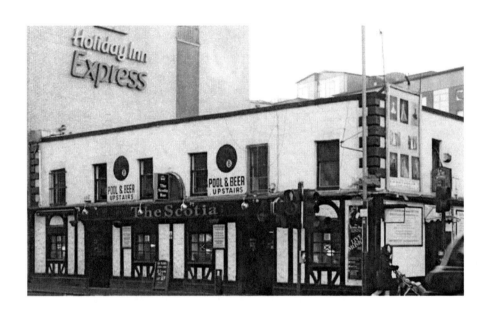

Glasglow's oldest pub

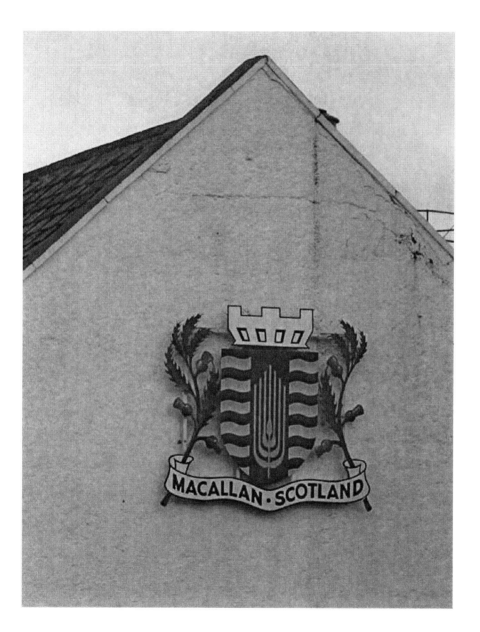

Scottish distillery

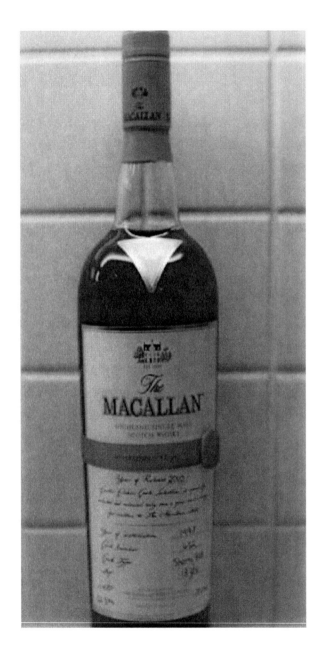

Best scotch I ever drank

Bawest Face in Scotland?

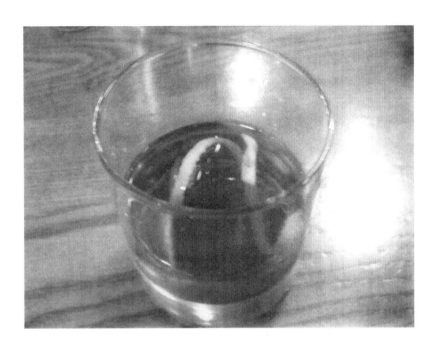

Best thing to do in New Orleans: Find the perfect Sezarac

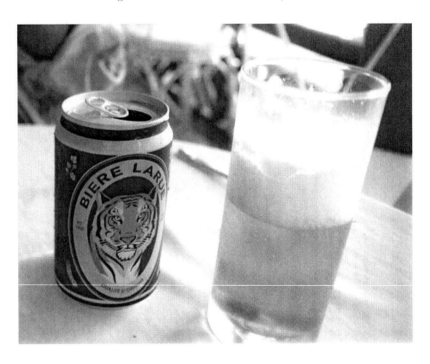

Viet Nam beer

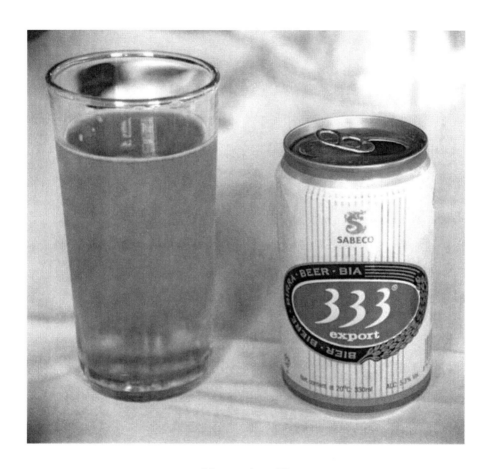

Viet nam beer #2

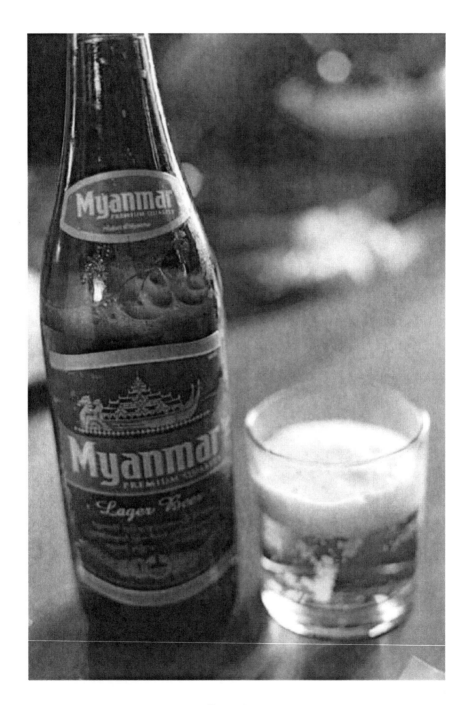

Burma beer

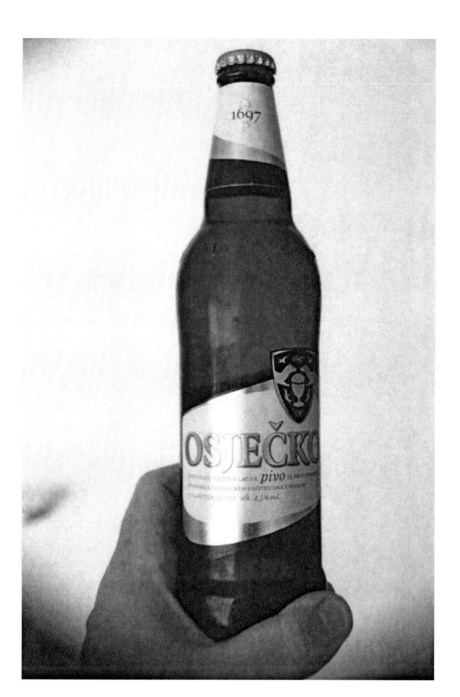

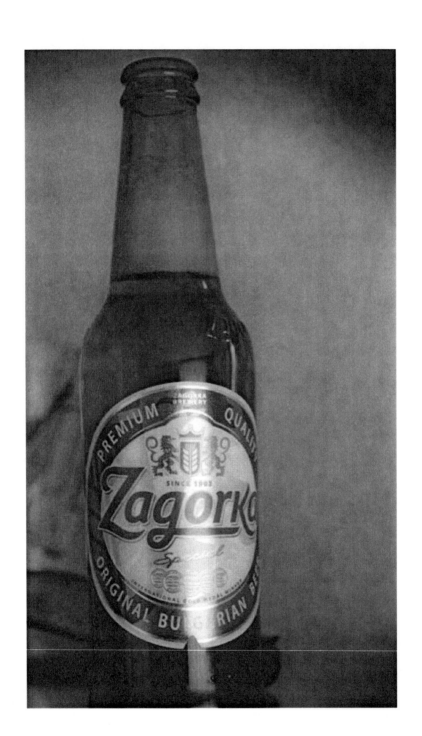

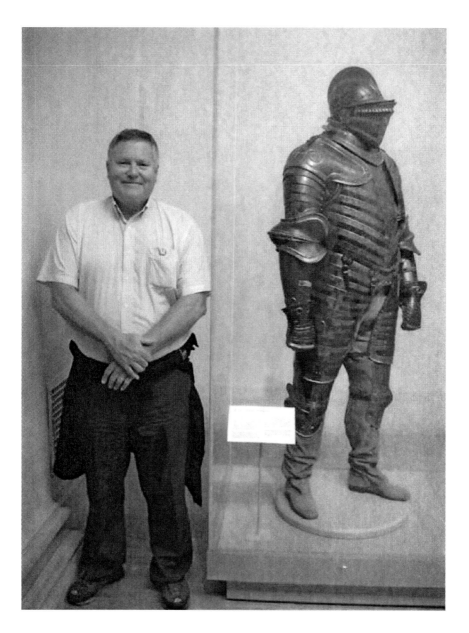

Henry the Eight looks like my genetic stock

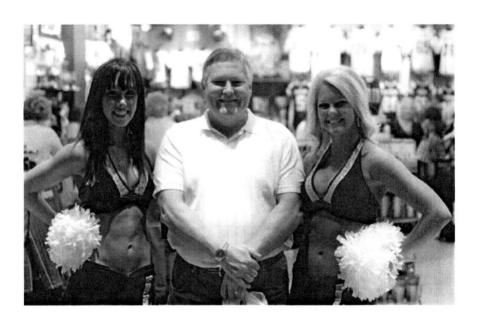

The day I became a Vikings fan. A tubby with two Twiggies.

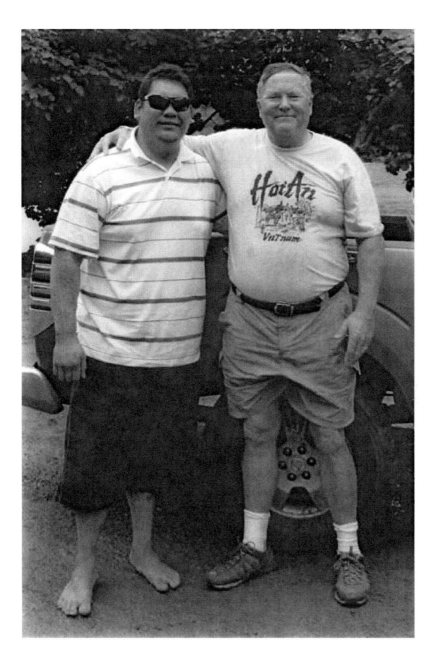

My French Polynesian Twin

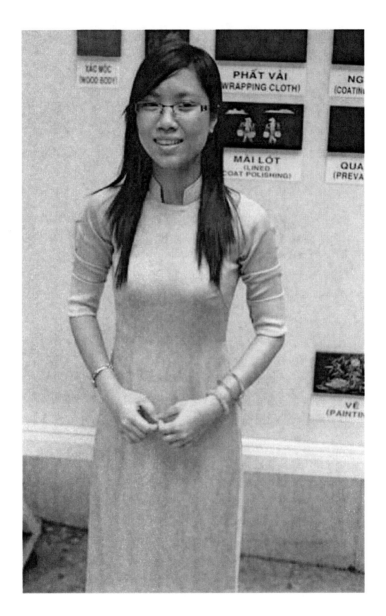

Vietnam prototype

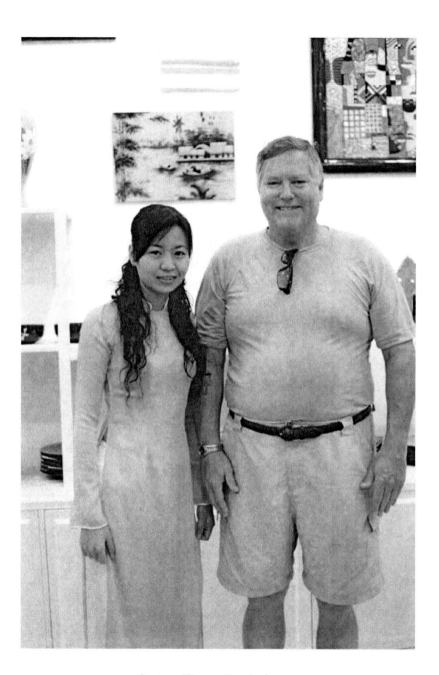

Contrast West vs. East body type

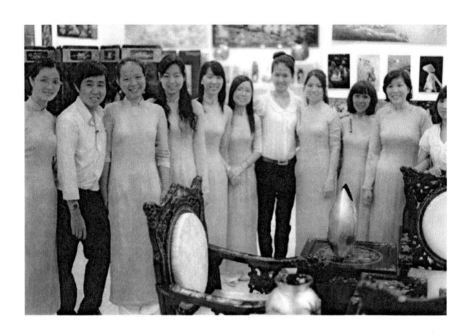

Genetic proof of thinness

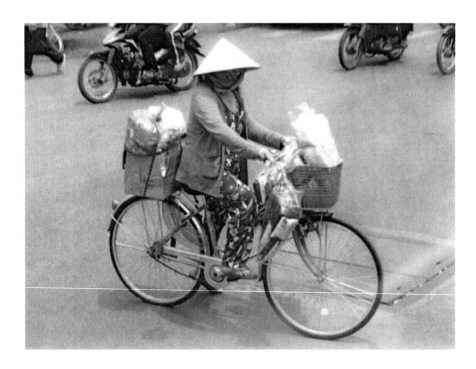

The cure to America's Obesity?

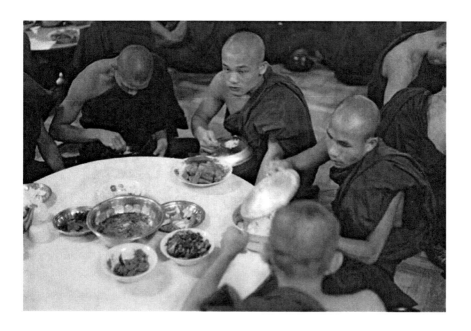

Burma Buddhist Buffett: 5% fat in diet

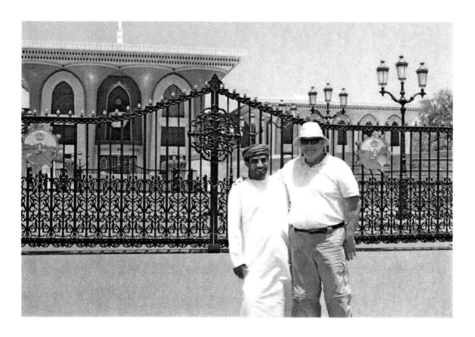

This is Oman. In Saudia Arabia there is an outbreak of obesity and type II Diabetes

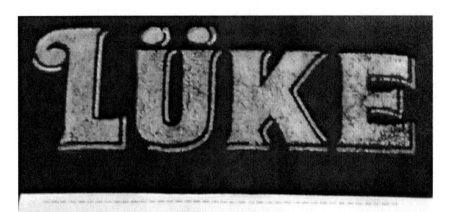

```
Tbl 72/1        Chk 1443           Gst 3
           Mar07'11 03:26PM
- - - - - - - - - - - - - - - - - - - - - - - - - -
       DINE IN
  3 SAZERAC                       13.50
  1 FRENCH 75                      4.75
 36 HAPPY P&J                     18.00
  1 BEET SALAD                     8.00
  1 BEEFEATER                      4.25
      Margarita
      Martini Rocks                1.00

   Food                           26.00
   Liquor                         23.50
   Tax                             4.83
   Total                      54.33
```

New Orleans

New Orleans

HERBSAINT
BAR AND RESTAURANT

```
0012  Table 41  #Party 3
TEAM 2 T    SvrCk:  4  5:56p 03/09/11


1 GUMBO                                 7.00
1 Antipasto                            12.00
1 SHRIMP CAKES                         11.00
1 JUMBO SHRIMP                         28.00
1 DUCK,JOINER                          27.00
1 SAZERAC                               9.00

                          Sub Total:   94.00
                               Tax:     9.17
                          Sub Total:  103.17
03/09  7:02p TOTAL:       103.17
```

New Orleans

New England Fish Market

Server: Brandi   02/21/2011
Table 34/2   2:38 PM
Guests: 4   20040

Cup New England Clam Ch   3.99
Cup Lob Bisque   4.99
Oysters Roccafeller   10.99
Fish Taco   3.99

Subtotal   23.96
Tax   1.56

Total   25.52

Balance Due   25.52

Ask your server for
a fish bucks card!

Jensen Beach, FL

Mythos-133

www.universalorlando.com

OPERATOR: Terrell T. 7596 TABLE NUMBER: 11
CHECK NUMBER: 1-65   GUEST COUNT: 6

TRX RESUMED 0005 0198
SUSPENDED ON 2/18/2011 12:51:41 PM

******* Stored Order *******

SEAT NUMBER 3
     Bistro Filet   15.95
     DIET COKE   2.25
SEAT NUMBER 5
     Fish Tacos   12.50
     ROMAINE CAESAR   6.75
     WATER W/ LEMON   0.00
     WG YELLOW TAIL   5.00

     SUBTOTAL   42.45
     18% Gratuity   7.64
     TAX   2.44
     AMOUNT DUE   52.53

Universal studio restaurant Mythos

```
DUBLIN CASTLE CAFE
***********************************
DATE 23/01/2011 SUN    TIME 15:15

DISH OF DAY 3              €7.50
SOUP BREAD                 €3.95
FLAV WATER                 €2.25
MINERAL                    €2.00
SUBTOTAL                  €15.70
TOTAL                     €15.70
CASH                      €50.00
CHANGE                    €34.30
CLERK 8          068706    00000
```

Ireland euro's

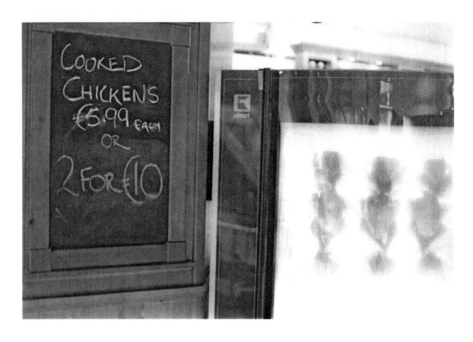

Roasted chicken is the best deal in most countries

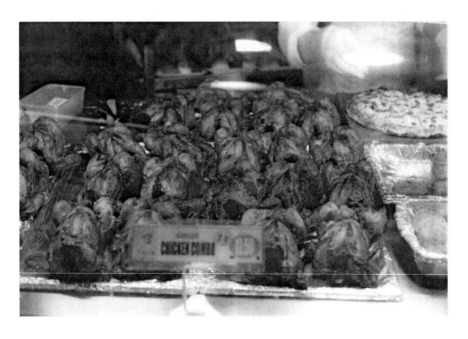

Roasted chicken in UAE

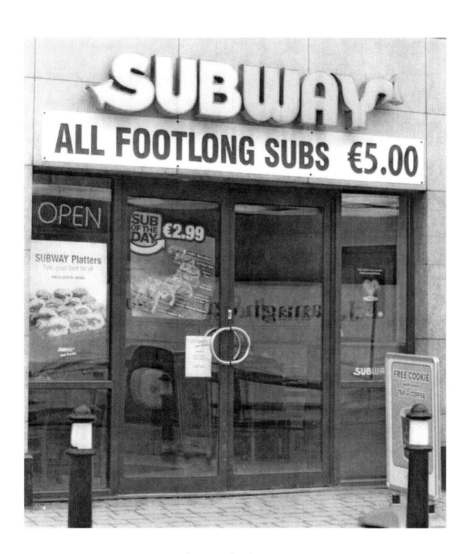

Ireland

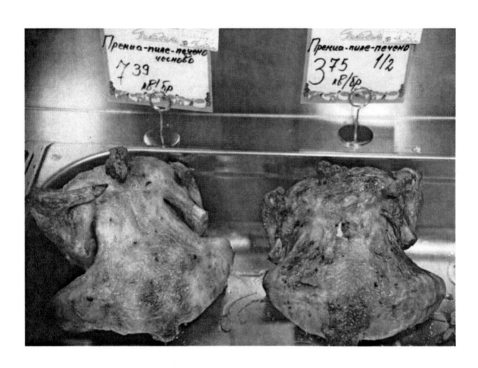

Roasted chicken tastes good everywhere

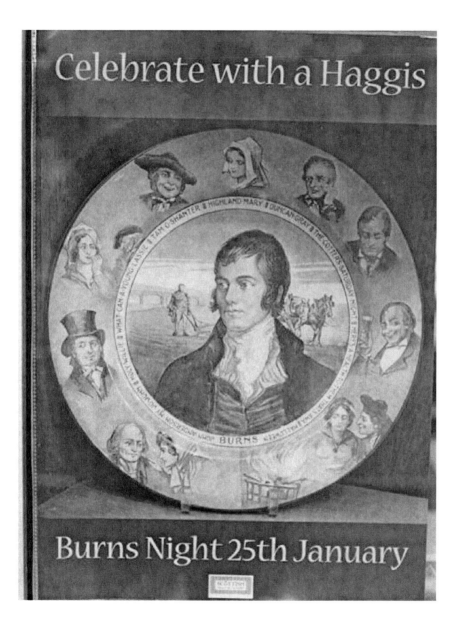

Celebrate with a Haggis

Burns Night 25th January

Haggis Scotland

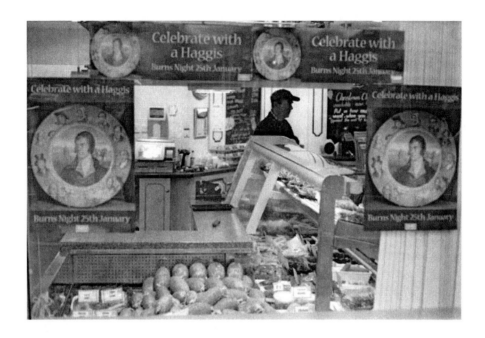

Scottish butcher

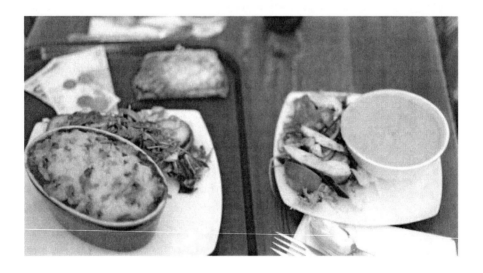

Irish Lunch

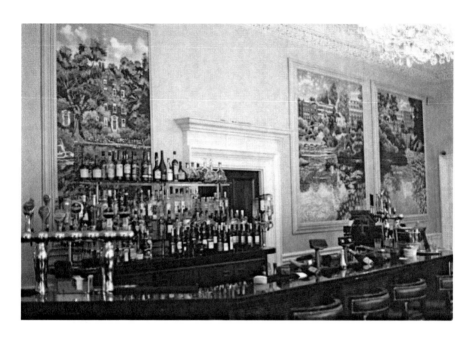

Shelborne Hotel bar in Dublin

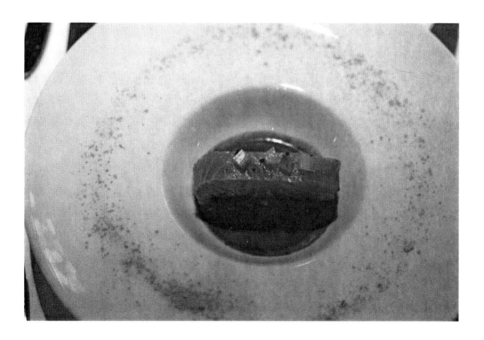

Prefect sashimi salmon in Dublin historical hotel, The Shelborne

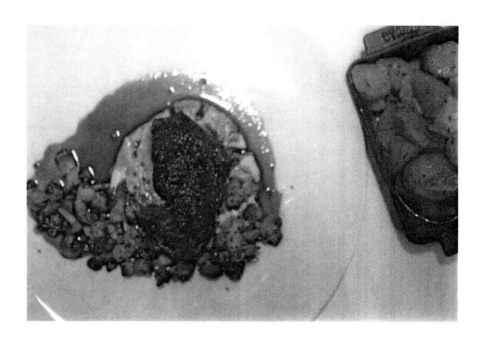

Shelborne lunch in Dublin

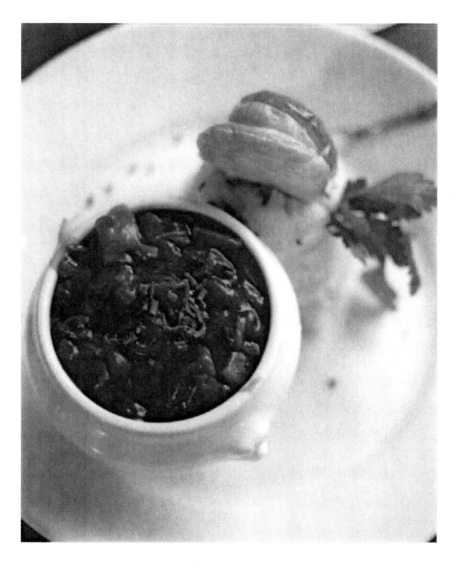

Guinness stew

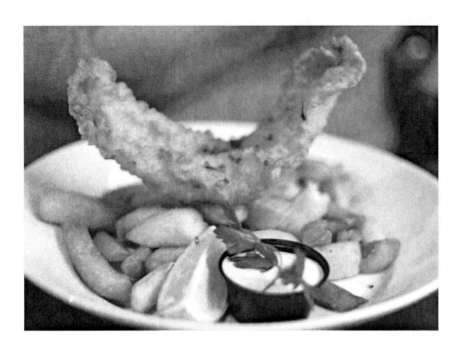

Fish and chips

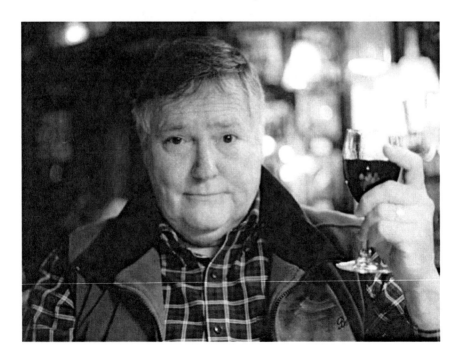

Hatties in Athelone, Ireland

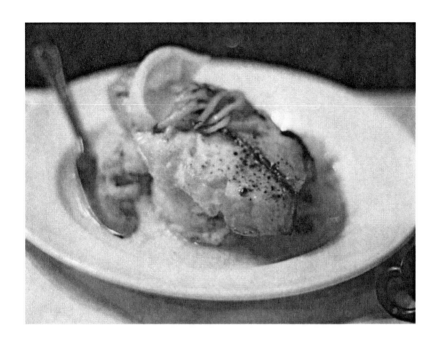

Hatties fish

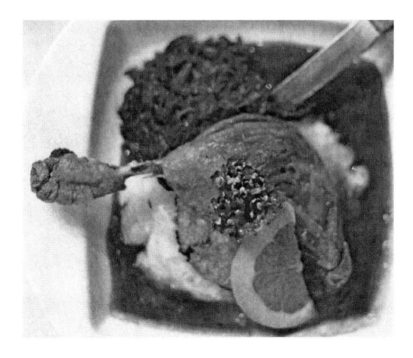

Duck confit at Hattie's

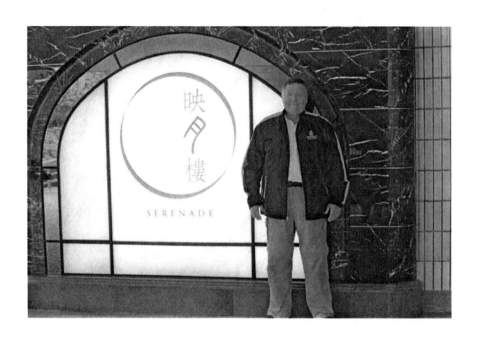

Hong Kong restaurant

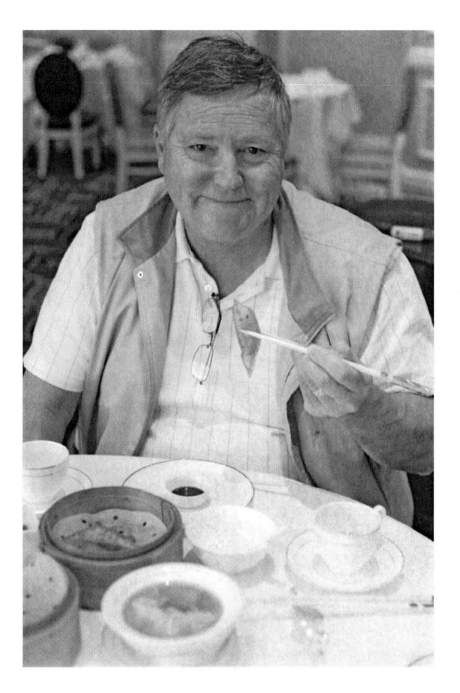

Dim Sum at Serenades

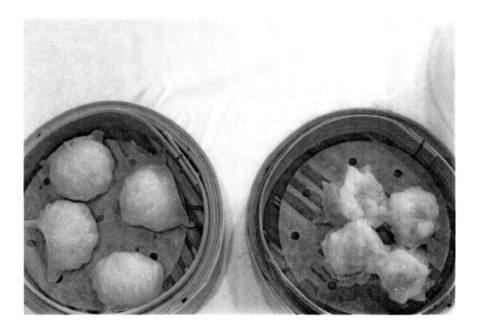

Serenade's Dim Sum

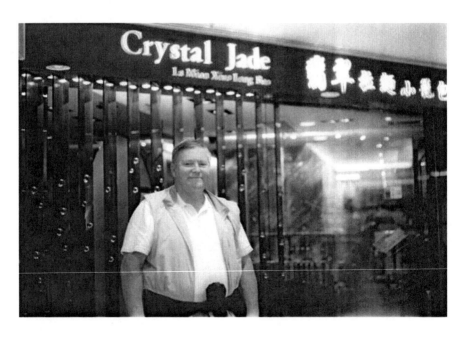

Good place for Dim Sum at the Mall in Hong Kong near the Star ferry. Get there early.

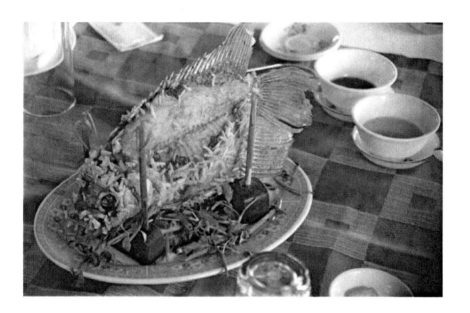

Fish on the Viet Nam delta

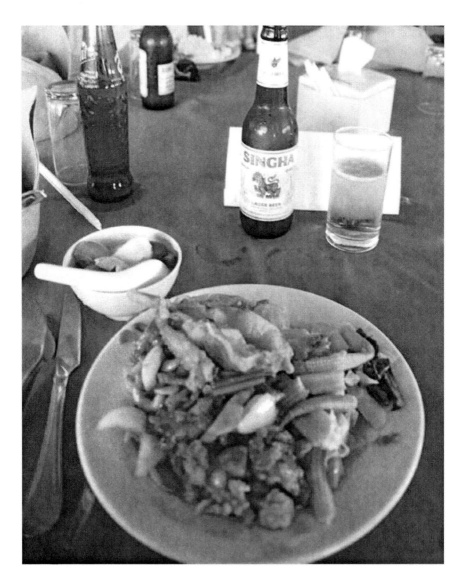

Buffett in Thailand

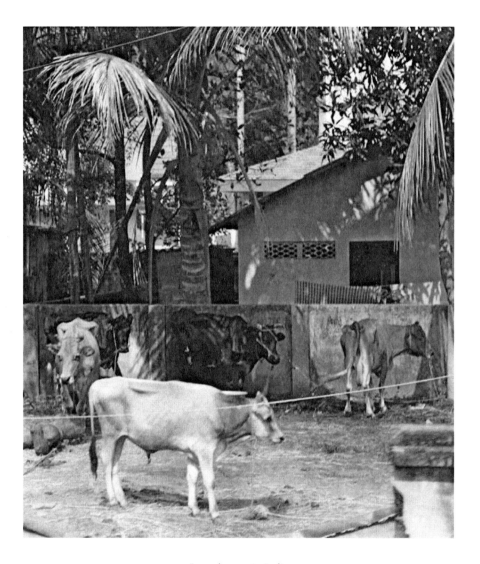

Sacred cows in India

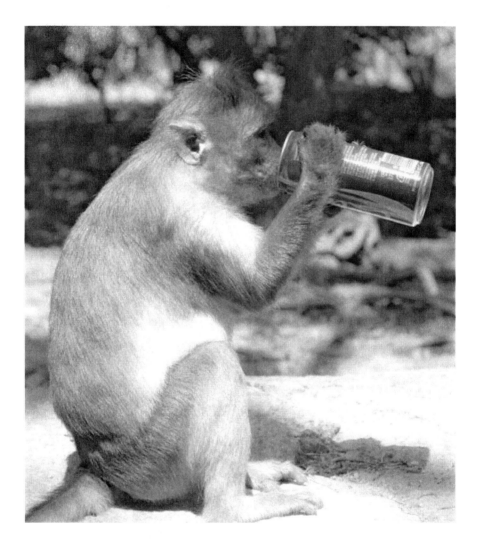

Monkey steals our Cola at Elephata Island, India

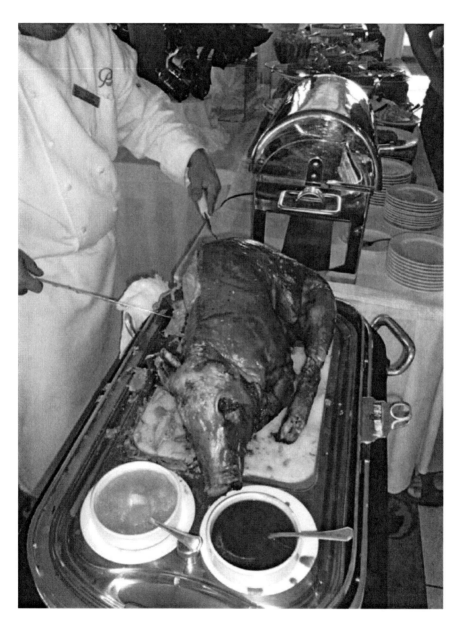

Polynesian pig on Paul Gauguin

Tubby Thought

"Luckily, with Time?"

"Sporadic bursts of activity, such as 'dieting,' are not effective; the behaviors that achieve and maintain a healthy body weight take a lifetime of commitment. Luckily, with time, these behaviors become second nature" (Nutrition: Concepts and Controversies [2011], p. 325).

Caveat emptor:

"Maybe the obese eat differently, gulping their food or skipping breakfast only to binge later in the day? But no, that also turned out not to be true. Some overweight people eat quickly, some slowly. Some binge, some do not. Some eat when they are stressed; some lose their appetites in those circumstances. And, in every case, thin people are just as likely as the obese to exhibit those behaviors. There is no behavior that is typical of the obese."

This conclusion was reached by Mickey Stunkard based on the Midtown Manhattan Trial 1962 as reported by Gina Kolata on page 93 in *Rethinking Thin* (2007).

Chapter 17

The History of Obesity and Diets

A Guide to Obesity and the Metabolic Syndrome: Origins and Treatment by George Bray, in the introduction and chapter 1.

Obesity is at least 30,000 years old as demonstrated in Eurasian artifacts.

"Diet and Exercise were the mainstays of treatment by Hippocrates."

"In 1847, while serving in the army, Helmholtz published his first masterpiece on the conservation of energy."

1973: Fenfluramine approved

1986: Vermont overfeeding study

1986: Twin overfeeding study

1992; Weintraub combined therapy

1994: Leptin gene cloned

The history of "fad" diet

The fattening carbohydrate from 1825 onward

Why We Get Fat: And What to Do about It by Gary Taubes

1. Brillat-Savarin wrote Physiologie du Gout (Physiology of Taste) in 1825.

Two principal causes of obesity:

1.1. "The natural constitution of the individual . . . some people, in whom the digestive forces manufacture, all things being equal, a greater supply of fat, as it were, destined to be obese."

1.2. Starches and flours and "starch produces this effect more quickly and surely when it is used with sugar."

2. Francois Dancel (1844)

    "I have established it as a fact, without single exception that it is always possible to diminish obesity, by living chiefly upon meat, and partaking only of a small quantity of other kinds of food."

3. Dr. William Harvey to Mr. Banting (1862)

    "It occurred to me . . . a combination of animal food with such vegetable diet as contained neither sugar or starch, might serve to arrest the undue formation of fat."

4. Mr. Banting, 1863: "A Letter on Corpulence" (translated around the world)

    In 1862, lost 50 lbs. on low-carb diet.

5. Thomas Tanner: *The Practice of Medicine* (1869)

    "The investigations pursued by Dr. Dancel having been mainly instrumental in leading to this result . . . Farinaceous (starchy) and vegetable foods are fattening, and saccharine matters are especially so."

6. Hilde Burch writes in her book *The Importance of Overweight* (1957) about a Congress of Internal Medicine in 1886:

    "The great progress in dietary control of obesity was the recognition that meat, the strong food, was not fat producing 'but that it was innocent foodstuffs, such as bread and sweets, which lead to obesity.'"

7. William Osler: *The Principles and Practice of Medicine* (1901)

    "In the case of women who tend to grow stout after child bearing or at the climacteric, in addition to systematic exercises, they should be told to avoid taking too much food, and particularly to reduce the starches and sugars."

8. James French: *A Text-Book on the Practice of Medicine* (1907)

"The principal causes that lead to (obesity) are excess of food and drink, especially of starches, sugars and malt liquors, with deficient exercise . . . The general indications are to reduce the quantity of carbohydrates ingested and the allowance of fluid; alcohol should be forbidden."

9. H. Gardiner Hill on "The Treatment of Obesity" in the Lancet (1925)

    "All forms of bread contain a large proportion of carbohydrate . . . It should thus be condemned."

10. A decade of diets for obesity that proposed low carbohydrates:

    1943: Stanford University School of Medicine
    1948: Harvard Medical School
    1950: Children's Memorial Hospital in Chicago
    1952: Cornell Medical School and New York Hospital

11. Raymond Greene: *The Practice of Endocrinology* (1951)

    His diet for obesity excluded carbohydrates and allowed as much as you like of meat, fish, foul, green vegetables, eggs, cheese, and fruit except bananas and grapes.

12. Dr. Spock: *Baby and Child Care* (six editions) (1946-1992)

    "The amount of plain, starchy foods taken is what determines, in the case of most people, how much (weight) they gain or lose."

13. Alfred Pennington: "Obesity in Industry–The Problem and Its Solution" (1949)

    Based on Blake Donaldson's diet: 1/2 lbs. of fatty meat for breakfast, lunch, and dinner, with one "hotel portion" of potato or fruit. No more than 80 carbohydrate calories at each meal. In a few cases, even this much carbohydrate prevented weight loss.

    Twenty obese DuPont executives lost between 9 lbs. and 54 lbs., averaging 3,000 calories a day.

14. George Thorpe: Kansas physician, chair of AMA's section of general practice in JAMA (1957):

"Evidence from widely different sources seems to justify the use of high-protein, high-fat, low-carbohydrate diets for successful loss of excess weight."

15. Hilde Bruch: *The Importance of Overweight* (1957)

She used the Pennington diet to help obese children lose weight.

16. Davidson and Passmore: *Human Nutrition and Dietetics* (1963)

"All popular slimming regimes involve a restriction in dietary carbohydrate."

17. Rosalyn Yalow and Soloman Berson, 1965, in Diabetes:

"Insulin is the principal regulator of fat metabolism and the release of fatty acids from fat cells requires only the negative stimulus of insulin deficiency."

18. George Cahill, coeditor of the American Physiological Society's Handbook of Physiology, section 5, "Adipose Tissue," sums it up this way:

"Carbohydrate is driving insulin is driving fat."

19. Edgar Gordon, JAMA 1963

"It may be stated categorically that the storage of fat, and therefore the production and maintenance of obesity, cannot take place unless glucose is being metabolized. Since glucose cannot be used by most tissues without the presence of insulin, it may also be stated categorically that obesity is impossible in the absence of adequate tissue concentrations of insulin ... Thus an abundant supply of carbohydrate food exerts a powerful influence in directing the stream of glucose metabolism into lipogenesis, whereas a relatively low carbohydrate intake tends to minimize the storage of fat."

This is the twelve-page article that Robert Atkins read and that led him to using a low-carbohydrate diet according to Gary Taubes.

20. Charlotte Young in an NIH conference: Obesity in Perspective (1973)

"In a series of carefully controlled metabolic studies ... carbohydrate-restricted diets gave excellent clinical results as measured by freedom from hunger, allaying of excessive fatigue, satisfactory weight loss, suitability for long term weight reduction and subsequent weight control . . . Weight loss, fat loss, and percent weight loss as fat appeared to be inversely related to the level of carbohydrate in the diets. No adequate explanation could be given for the differences in weight losses. Any of the low-carbohydrate diets used were effective in controlling hunger."

21. Consumer Reports magazine article on rating the diets, 1974

"The difficult-to-treat obese patient appears to suffer from some defect in dealing with carbohydrate which leads to an unnatural conversion of it to fat and to storage of the fat. Avoidance of too much dietary carbohydrate reduces this tendency."

I believe this defect is insulin resistance. The metabolic syndrome causes tubby patients to produce a higher-than-normal level of insulin in response to eating carbohydrates. This excess insulin causes the rapid conversion of the carbohydrates to fat.

The beauty of this lecture by Gary Taubes is the demonstration that Atkins diet is not a fad or bizarre. He then explains how this paradigm was changed to the low-fat paradigm. What is amazing is that this change occurred based on very little evidence-based medicine. It changed because of eminence-based medicine. The eminent Ancel Keys and Dr. Jean Mayer were very instrumental in changing the paradigm from low-carbohydrate to low-fat because of the belief that high-fat diets cause heart disease. The six-nation trial and then the seven-nation trial were the studies that proved their point. Unfortunately, we now realize the data was cooked to the outcome that was desired. It is a sad commentary on modern science.

1. *New York Times* article on July 7, 1965, by William Borders: "New diet decried by nutritionists. Dangers are seen in low carbohydrate intake."

The danger was the increase in fat resulting from the decrease in carbohydrate. This raised concern of more heart disease. Thus the statement, "It is the fat increase that prompted Dr. Jean Mayer of Harvard to say that encouraging the diet for middle aged Americans is, 'in a sense, equivalent to mass murder."

2. Dr. Robert Atkins published his book in 1971.

There was a response in a statement of American Medical Association Council on Foods and Nutrition in 1973:

Carbohydrate-restricted diets are "bizarre concepts of nutrition and dieting (that) should not be promoted to the public as if they were established scientific principles."

In the lecture, Gary Taubes goes on to say that Atkins was criticized for claiming there was a fat-mobilizing hormone. Gary Taubes states that "every hormone is fat mobilizing except insulin. The other hormones cannot mobilize the fat if insulin is elevated."

The critics said there was not a single unique fat-mobilizing hormone and that fat is mobilized when insulin levels are low.

This is on slide 36 of Gary Taubes's lecture. If it is true, it goes to show that there was more interest in attacking Dr. Atkins than trying to understand the truth.

3. Senator George McGovern, Report of the Select Committee on Nutrition and Human Needs, U.S. Senate, 1977

    Dietary Goals for the United States
    a. Increase carbohydrate consumption to account for 55-60% of the energy (caloric) intake.
    b. Reduce overall fat consumption from approximately 40 to 30% of energy intake.

    This is the document that officially changed the paradigm.

4. Jane Brody wrote in 1981 in the *Nutrition Book*:

    "We need to eat more carbohydrates."

5. Jane Brody's *Good Food Book: Living the High-Carbohydrate Way* in 1985:

    "Not only is eating pasta at the height of fashion, it can help you lose weight."

6. W. P. James et al.: *Proposals for Nutritional Guidelines for Health Education in Britain* (1983)

    "The previous nutritional advice in the UK to limit the intake of all carbohydrates as a means of weight control now runs counter to current thinking."

7.   The American Heart Association 1995 pamphlet:

      "To control the amount of and kind of fat, saturated fatty acids and dietary
      cholesterol you eat, choose snacks from other food groups such as . . . low-fat
      cookies, low-fat crackers . . . unsalted pretzels, hard candy, gum drops, sugar,
      syrup, honey, jam, jelly, marmalade (as spreads)."

8.   The USDA food pyramid called for carbohydrates as the largest portion of our
      food intake.

      On slide 42 of Gary Taubes's talk, he shows a table of the NHANES percentage
      of fat people in the USA. It jumped from 16% to 23% during the time of the
      paradigm shift from low-carb diets to low-fat diets. It begs the question, did the
      nutritionists and George McGovern cause the obesity epidemic?

Tubby Thought

Fat People Have Immoral Behavior? Gluttony?

"Despite increased awareness and behavioral treatment advances, the worldwide prevalence of obesity and weight-related chronic illnesses continues to expound. Behavioral treatment is inherently challenging and time-consuming, and readily available only to a fraction of the population who may benefit from inclusion. Several investigators have cautioned that individual or group-based interventions are insufficient to serve the population masses requiring treatment . . ."

Brent Van Dorsten, PhD, and Emily M. Lindley, PhD
Med Clin N Am, 95(2011), pp. 971-988.
Sept. 2011. Number 5.

Chapter 18

Old Game Plan

Cut your calories by 500 calories a day, walk thirty minutes a day. Lose a pound a week? So easy.

Yes, it is easy in the short term. This is why any diet that does this will work in the short term. It might work long term if you only lose 5% of your weight.

If you are 200 lbs. before the diet, you should stop the diet after you lose 10 lbs. Afterward you should weigh yourself every day, and if you gain three to 5 lbs., you must have a plan that you will immediately implement.

I think this is a very reasonable plan for people who don't need to lose 20% of their body weight to be healthy in terms of glucose, blood pressure, and the ability to pursue an exercise program. If you lose more than 8% of your body weight, you may decrease your exercise metabolism to 42% less. You may also hit your leptin threshold. This means your brain will want you to get fatter. It will increase anabolism of fat. It will put you on a more efficient energy expenditure. I call this the Sponge Syndrome.

What does this mean? It means that after one to five years, only 5% of the dieters will not gain back most of their weight. Despite this fact, the false hope goes on.

No one knows what to do when a reduced obese person hits his plateau other than continue a substarvation diet for at least one to two more years in the hope that his EE (energy expenditure) will become less efficient and he will lose some of his shrunken fat cells.

There are 6,000 people listed in the National Weight Control Registry who have succeeded at this. Apparently, many of these people have had a major change in their life. They recently divorced or changed their jobs. They also exercise not just to lose weight but because they get other benefits from it. They are also special people. They weigh themselves every day. If they gain three to 5 lbs., they know exactly what they need to do to lose the weight, and they do it. They are highly motivated. They are capable of cognitive restructuring. This means they replace negative thoughts with positive thoughts. They even have the energy and motivation to write it all down; the food, the activity, their feelings, and the positive thoughts they need to replace the negative thoughts they have every thirty minutes of the day. They are satisfied with a diet that does not have much variety.

When I lost 80 lbs. and hit the plateau after about fifteen months, I was cold all the time. I wanted to lose another 10 lbs. I decided to gain more muscle to improve my metabolism. I exercised two to three hours a day. I ate more fruit as I thought that was healthy food with antioxidants. I drank more alcohol. Three and a half years after I hit the plateau, I had gained back 58 lbs. I had retired thirteen months before and had increased my exercise even more. I went to water aerobics three mornings a week. I had two trainers working with me twice a week, each training session done in addition to my usual hour of exercise in the morning. The trainers did get me to a much higher intensity level and improved my core strength. I still gained half a pound each week on the average.

On January 1, 2011, I read *Why We Get Fat: And What to Do about It* by Gary Taubes. This brought me to a new game plan:

For tubby people with metabolic syndrome, go on a low-carbohydrate diet.

For people with CC genotype, it seems they do better with low-fat diet. Ornish diet seems extremely difficult to me, but vegans seem to have a whole lifestyle change that they embrace. Beware that being a vegan does not mean you can eat all the low-fat dessert you want. The Southeast Asians are vegetarians. The Southeast Asians in America have been described as being "contaminated vegetarians." They do very badly with metabolic syndrome and cardiovascular disease.

If you look at the recent trials (i.e., Gardner and Sachs), the low-fat group and the low-carb group usually start to gain back weight after six months. Is this because of the plateau? Or is it due to noncompliance? It is clear that they did not follow the diets carefully. They both drifted to more fat in the low fat group and more carbohydrates in the low carbohydrate group.

Both Ornish and Atkins allow you to eat all that you want. This is why I advise one or the other. You must follow a diet that gives you satiety! Once you have satiety, you are much more likely to comply with on the diet in the long term. Walk at least ten minutes a day. Do not do any exercise program you will not stay on for the rest of your life. I don't want you to lose a lot of weight rapidly. I also don't want you to injure yourself. Once you walk at least ten minutes a day, you have achieved most of the health benefits of exercise. If you don't lose weight on this diet, don't be discouraged. As long as you don't gain weight and you don't feel hungry, you are on the right track. I did not lose weight on my low-carb diet. I decreased my exercise because I was traveling so much. I was just happy I ate as much as I wanted, and I didn't gain weight. For the first time in my life I was not hungry between meals. The 30 g of protein with each meal has provided satiety. A big problem for the eat-all-you-want dieters is to realize that you should eat not to the point of feeling stuffed. You need to learn to eat to the point of being full. It was difficult for me to do that, but I think I finally did get to that point the eight month into my very low-carbohydrate diet.

I am amazed that I have been on several cruises, I decreased my overall exercise, and I ate 60% fat, my cholesterol is good; and I don't feel deprived. I feel as if I can stay on this diet for the rest of my life.

Get CAC and CIMT at the start of the program. Get LDL-P at the start of the program and every four months. Have your doctor check your blood pressure every four months. If you have a blood pressure problem, you should have a cuff at home and check it each morning. If you have diabetes type II, follow your glucose each morning and get your Hgb A1C four times a year. Repeat your CAC in five years and repeat your CIMT in two to three years.

Tubby Thought

Twenty-Two Pounds of Inevitable Fat

"Over 30 years, the daily ingestion of only 8 kcal more than expended can increase body weight by 10 kg. This represents the average amount of weight gained by Americans during the 30-year period between 25 and 55 years of age." p. 1607

Williams Textbook of Endocrinology, 2011, 12th edition by Shlomo Melmed et al.

Saunders Elsevier referenced from Rosenbaum M. et al., Obesity. N Engl J Med 1997; 337-408.

Caveat emptor:

"Older people have a lower metabolic expenditure than younger ones and as a rule lose weight more slowly since metabolic rates decline by approximately 2% per decade (about 100 kcal per decade) (Lin et al. 2003)" (George A. Bray, *A Guide to Obesity and the Metabolic Syndrome: Origins and Treatment* [CRC Press, 2011], p. 179).

Chapter 19

The Reduced Obese

I am at the Obesity Society meeting in Orlando. The science of obesity has exploded. The problem is extremely complex. It's all about treating the reduced obese or weight loss maintenance. No one knows the answers. The FDA has shot down the last four diet pills. Combination diet pills will be the answer in the future. The problem is that 60% of the U.S. population will take the pills. That means many pregnant women may take it by accident. The last diet pill had to pay out $2 billion in damages. In the meantime, it is bariatric surgery that is saving lives. Our society seems to feel there is a moral hazard to simply take a pill to lose weight, while an expensive and dangerous surgery is acceptable?

The Reduced Obese

This is the problem. The problem is not what is the best diet. The problem is not low-fat vs. low-carb diet. The problem is how do you not regain weight once you lose it. There is no solution right now. In the future there will be combination medication and prevention with genetic and phenotype screening for babies. Prevention is the solution but we do not have a clue how to do this right now.

I am a member of the Reduced Obese. In my particular case, I have stopped gaining weight by going on a very low-carbohydrate diet in the year of 2011. If you are tubby or have the metabolic syndrome (which means you are insulin resistant), you should try to stay on a low-carbohydrate diet.

However, there are clearly obese people who do not respond to low-carbohydrate diets. These people are probably not insulin resistant and perhaps have a CC genotype.

An insulin resistant patient may have lost weight with a low-carb diet but then when he loses 50 lbs.; he may no longer be insulin resistant and the low-carbohydrate diet may not work as well.

More importantly, the patient fell off the obese EE (energy expenditure) curve down to a more efficient EE curve that burns calories very slowly. The patient has hit his resettlement point or plateau and the leptin plateau or leptin threshold is reached. The patient becomes hungry, slows metabolism, and anabolism of fat occurs. I call this the Sponge Syndrome. It's as if you are winning at poker and suddenly you find yourself playing blackjack. The rules change.

The key to all this is satiety. I found satiety with 30 g of protein per meal with three meals a day, high-fat diet and low-carbohydrate diet. This gives me the time to learn to not overeat.

It is not about hypocalorie diets and *exercise.* Diet and exercise programs have, and will, fail because of the *reduced obese problem.*

Look at the people who have succeeded. The National Weight Control Registry has a list of 6,000 people who have succeeded. God bless them and God have mercy on them. In the Obesity Issue of Medical Clinics of North American Sept. 2011 on p. 945, Dubnov-Raz and Berry write, "Both men and women (in the NWCR) consumed a low-fat diet (24%) and exercised to use 470 to 360 calories kcal/d, respectively. The net energy balance was 918 kcal/d for women and 1225 kcal/for men. These reduced obese subjects ate an average of five meals a day and conducted a very regimented existence."

Every commercial diet program must have a disclaimer at the bottom of their advertisement. *If* this product is successful you will become one of the *reduced obese.* Adverse effects of this condition:

1. The leptin threshold (plateau or settling point) will be reached.
2. This will make you more hungry, decrease your metabolism and cause you to make more fat.
3. It will take you off your high calorie expending physiology (EE) and knock you over to a new energy expending physiology that will force you to be on a

very low-calorie, high exercise product for one to two years to get rid of many of the adiposites that make the leptin and allow you to return to your previous energy expenditure physiology.

4. The result of being on this substarvation diet may scar your psyche similar to concentration camp internees. (see Ancel Keys study)

Tubby Thought

Mass Murder!

"Encouraging the diet (low carbohydrate) in middle aged Americans is in a sense equivalent to mass murder."

Dr. Jean Mayer of Harvard, leading nutritionist in America
July 7, 1965, taken from Gary Taubes's book, *Why We Get Fat: And What to Do about It.*

Caveat emptor:

The A-Z trial and the comparative diet trial both showed the Atkins diet to be lipid neutral and thus safe.

1. Gardner CD et al., Comparison of the Atkins, Zone, Ornish, and LEARN Diets for Change in Weight and Related Risk Factors Among Overweight Premenopausal Women: The A to Z Weight Loss Study: A Randomized Trial. JAMA. 2007 Mar 7; 297(9):969-77. *http://www.ncbi.nlm.nih.gov/entrez/query.fcgi?db=PubMed&cmd=Retrieve&list_uids=17341711&dopt=Abstract* [PMID: 17341711]
    King DE et al., Adherence to Healthy Lifestyle Habits in US Adults, 1988-2006. Am J Med., 2009 Jun; 122(6):528-34. *http://www.ncbi.nlm.nih.gov/entrez/query.fcgi?db=PubMed&cmd=Retrieve&list_uids=19486715&dopt=Abstract* [PMID: 19486715]

2. Sachs FM et al., Comparison of Weight-Loss Diets with Different Compositions of Fat, Protein, and Carbohydrates. N Engl J Med., 2009 Feb 26; 360(9):859-73. *http://www.ncbi.nlm.nih.gov/entrez/query.fcgi?db=PubMed&cmd=Retrieve&list_uids=19246357&dopt=Abstract* [PMID: 19246357]

Chapter 20

The Great Fat Debate

This debate occurred on November 8, 2010:

Q: "The scientific advisory report . . . talks about a more plant-based diet . . . that could end up being a higher carbohydrate diet."

Dr. Willett: "Just being plant-based doesn't necessarily mean it's going to be healthy . . . In general moving toward a plant-based diet will be healthier. For example replacing red meat with some combination of nuts and legumes."

(I find it interesting that Dr. Willett made this statement when his colleague, Dr. Mozaffarian, published an article about red meat in Circulation whose conclusion states, "Consumption of processed meats but not red meats, is associated with higher incidence of CVD." This article was received on November 25, 2009, and accepted on April 8, 2010.)

Dr. Lichenstein: "We have to be careful about simplifying messages too much, because we may end up with unanticipated consequences. I think that's what happened with the low-fat message, which contributed to an increase in sugar and refined carbohydrate intakes."

(Am. J Clin Nutr 2007; 86(3): 707-13. This was an eighteen-month randomized trial of a low-glycemic index diet and weight change in Brazilian women. Two hundred eight women were on two diets with 41-point difference in glycemic index. They did not have a significant difference in weight loss. No differences in hunger. To replace fat with fruits and vegetables does not seem to make a difference [as opposed to sugar and refined carbohydrates].)

A low glycemic might be defined as < 50
Potato, white, baked in skin 85
Whole wheat bread (one slice) 77
Bran flakes cereal 74
Popcorn, microwaved 72
Pineapple, diced 66
Oatmeal instant, cooked 66
Raisins 64
Beets, canned 64
Figs, dried 61
Corn, sweet, boiled 60
Granulated table sugar (sucrose) 68
Brown sugar 59
Kiwi fruit 58
Apricots 57
Banana 52

I tried to eat healthy, by eating:
Apples 38
Avocados 0
Cherries, sweet with pits 22
Grapes, green 46
Pears 38

(I ate fruit every day. I had a salad every day with Newman's balsalmic vinaigrette. I gained 58 lbs. over four years despite two hours of exercise a day.)

Q: "True or false—is saturated fat artery-clogging?"

Dr. Kuller: "It's not 7% (saturated fat), which makes atherosclerosis, it's what it does to apoB or LDL cholesterol."

Dr. Willett: "Replacing saturated fat with fine starch and sugar will not reduce the cardiovascular risk."

Dr. Mozaffarian: "Compared with polyunsaturated fats (vegetable oils), saturated fat is harmful; compared with the average carbohydrate consumed saturated fat is neutral; compared with refined starches and sugars, saturated fat may actually be relatively beneficial in many individuals."

Dr. Kuller: "I'll say that what you just said is wrong . . . I can show you unequivocally that among diabetics, to prevent heart disease, you've got to lower the LDL-C or the apoB and not primarily lowering the blood glucose . . . you do that (lower LDL-C), basically, by giving a statin."

Dr. Lichenstein: "We need to give guidance about what (to replace fat with) . . . (for example) displace butter with soft margarine rather than an extra slice of toast, omit cheese on salad with oil and vinegar rather than adding fat-free salty croutons"

Q: "Are n6 fatty acids inflammatory?"

Dr. Willett: "N6s are not proinflammatory."

Dr. Mozaffarian: "Agreed."

Dr. Lichtenstein: "Agreed."

Q: "(Is) the LDL particle size, the small, dense particles, being a higher risk for heart disease versus the large?"

Dr. Kuller: "LDL size has almost no importance."

Reference: *Journal of the American Dietetic Association*, May 2011, volume 111, number 5, pp. 672-675.

Participants:
On November 8, 2010
Walter C. Willett, MD, DrPH, Harvard
Fredrick John Stare Professor of Epidemiology and Nutrition Chair, Department of Nutrition
http://www.hsph.harvard.edu/departments/epidemiology/
Department of Epidemiology
Boston, Massachusetts
The primary studies conducted by our group involve several large ongoing prospective cohorts: the 121,700-member Nurses' Health Study, initiated by Dr. Frank Speizer at the Channing Laboratory; the Health Professionals Follow-up Study, a cohort of 52,000 men; and the Nurses' Health Study II, a cohort of younger women numbering 116,000

Dietary data have been collected from all of these populations, including seven cycles in the Nurses' Health Study.

Lewis K. Kuller, MD, DrPH, Distinguished University Professor of Public Health
Department of Epidemiology, University of Pittsburgh.
Pittsburgh, PA 15213
kullerl@edc.pitt.edu
Epidemiology of Cardiovascular Risk Factors in Women (1983-2012) NHLBI
Cardiovascular Health Study Events Follow Up (2005-2010) University of Washington
Clinical Trial / Observational Study of the Women's Health Initiative (WHI) (2005-2010) NHLBI
Hormone Therapy, Estrogen Metabolism and Risk in the WHI (2007-2009) NHLBI
Reduction of Triglycerides in Women on Hormone Therapy (2007-2009)
Ginkgo Biloba Prevention Trial in Older Adults (2005-2010)
Rheumatoid Arthritis and Risk of CVD and Total Mortality
Epidemiology of Heterogeneity in type 2 Diabetes
Epidemiology of Putative Genuine Genetic Variants: The WHI

Dariush Mozafarian, MD, DrPH
Associate Professor in the Department of Epidemiology
http://www.hsph.harvard.edu/departments/epidemiology
Department of Epidemiology
Boston, Massachusetts
dmozaffa@hsph.harvard.edu

Alice H. Lichtenstein DSc
Senior Scientist and Director
http://www.hnrc.tufts.edu/1192109687036/HNRCA-Page-
Cardiovascular Nutrition Laboratory
Jean Mayer USDA HNRCA at Tufts University
Boston, MA

Tubby Thought

The Reduced Obese Are Doomed to a Substarvation State

"Ancel Keys had men of normal weight go on a weight loss diet. Their metabolism slowed by 40%. They became fixated on food. They act like people from the WWII concentration camps.

Jules Hirsch found the obese had numerous and huge fat cells. People who lost 100 pounds look like someone who was never fat but they are different. By every measurement they seemed liked people who were starving" (Gina Kolata, *Rethinking Thin*).

Caveat emptor:

If you are a tubby by nature, beware of the current guidelines that push diet and exercise first. Only 6,000 people are documented by NWCR to have maintained weight loss for more than five years. These people are living in a substarvation state. Are you prepared to do that for the rest of your life?

Chapter 21

Caveat emptor:

There is a great deal of confusion in diet books about what a healthy diet is and what is a good cholesterol level. This book is a call for a new look at old ideas.

1. There is a cholesterol saturation point. You can't avoid eating less than 200 mg of cholesterol, and eating more than 300 mg doesn't seem to make a difference, so why worry about it?
2. Turns out red meat is safe–a sea change at Harvard.
3. Processed meats have a lot of salt, but if you are on a low-carb diet, you need more salt unless you are salt sensitive.
4. Replacing unsaturated fats with carbs was a big mistake. Another sea change at Harvard.
5. Ancel Keys choose the data that fitted his lipid hypothesis. He was the father of the "low-fat diet" movement. Old articles use old terminology. They will write that low-fat diets cause lower total cholesterol. Part of that is because it lowers good cholesterol and raises triglycerides.

Demand that writers write in modern terms.

1. LDL-P not LDL-C.
2. HDL-P not HDL-C.
3. If not LDL-P then apoB or the Tubby Factor (non-HDL cholesterol).
4. Forget ratios (i.e., HDL to total cholesterol).

5. A diet has to state outcomes after five years at a minimum.
6. The reduced obese state must be addressed in every diet
7. Look at the date of the references.
8. In the diets, is there a subset for genetic types and metabolic syndrome?

Truth:
If you get your LDL-P to 750, there is very little inflammation.
The CRPhs, triglycerides, and HDL don't matter once the LDL-P goal is reached.

The blood pressure and glucose is important and no smoking.

Weight loss usually makes everything better, but only 5% of people maintain their weight loss for five years.

In October, I went online to chat with other believers in the low-carb diet. Unfortunately, this group of people are statin adverse.

They cite the book the *Cholesterol Myth* by Malcolm Kendrick, MD. I was reading this 2007 edition, and the information seemed ancient. I went online and found a 2009 Jimmy Moore interview with Dr. Kendrick. I give him great credit for challenging the views of saturated fat and cholesterol in the diet. He clearly said on the interview that if you have heart disease, you should clearly take a statin if you can tolerate it. It will decrease cardiovascular events. Somehow that message was lost on many Fat Head fans. However, I can understand the confusion. Dr. Kendrick, in his book the *Great Cholesterol Con*, on page 168, pulls three important facts together:

1. Fact one: Statins do not reduce overall mortality in women.
2. Fact two: Statins do not reduce overall mortality in men without heart disease.
3. Fact three: Statins do not, therefore, reduce mortality in more than 95% of the adult population.

Caveat emptor: The copyright for this information is 2007.

In 2009, Dr. Kendrick was interviewed on the Jimmy Moore show

This is for people who are statin adverse. Dr. Kendrick advises taking statins for people with MIs or at high risk in this interview in 2009. It is a change from what he seemed to write in his book in 2007.

http://www.thelivinlowcarbshow.com/shownotes/271/dr-malcom-kendrick-debunks-the-
Dr. Malcolm Kendrick Debunks *The Great Cholesterol Con* (Episode 263)
http://www.thelivinlowcarbshow.com/
www.thelivinlowcarbshow.com

Jimmy shares his recent discussion with Dr. Malcolm Kendrick, author of *The Great Cholesterol Con*. Dr. Kendrick raises the inconvenient truths that science does not support the highly-touted cholesterol theory behind heart disease and that there is no such thing as "blood cholesterol."

In the interview, Dr. Kendrick answers the question, "What is good about statins?" Statins decrease death from cardiovascular or coronary artery disease. No one can deny that. Statins decrease risk of cardiovascular disease. In people with a heart attack or at high risk, it probably is a good idea to take a statin if you don't have side effects.

Tubby Thought

Energy Expenditure

Ethan Sims did a study to get college students to gain weight. He failed. He then used prisoners of normal weight to force them to gain weight. He succeeded. It took four to six months and up to 10,000 calories a day to get them to gain 25 lbs. The prisoners metabolism increased by 50%. The prisoners' fat cells grew larger but not more in number. After the study the prisoners had no trouble losing the weight.

Rethinking Thin, Gina Kolata

Caveat emptor:

The argument that the first law of thermodynamics applies equally to all in the realm of obesity is flawed. There is a tubby world and a twiggy world with different biology and genetics that process calories in the form of carbohydrates, fats, and protein in different ways and rates.

Chapter 22

Gardner and Sachs Trial

Gardner Trial

JAMA. 2007 Mar 7; 297(9):969-77.
Comparison of the Atkins, Zone, Ornish, and LEARN Diets for Change in Weight and Related Risk Factors Among Overweight Premenopausal Women: The A to Z Weight Loss Study: A Randomized Trial. Gardner CD, Kiazand A, Alhassan S, Kim S, Stafford RS, Balise RR, Kraemer HC, and King AC.

Source: Stanford Prevention Research Center and the Department of Medicine, Stanford University Medical School, Stanford, California, USA.

cgardner@stanford.edu
Erratum in JAMA. 2007 Jul 11; 298(2):178.

Abstract

Context:

Popular diets, particularly those low in carbohydrates, have challenged current recommendations advising a low-fat, high-carbohydrate diet for weight loss. Potential benefits and risks have not been tested adequately.

Objective:

To compare four weight-loss diets representing a spectrum of low to high carbohydrate intake for effects on weight loss and related metabolic variables.

Design, Setting, and Participants:

Twelve-month randomized trial conducted in the United States from February 2003 to October 2005 among 311 free-living, overweight/obese (body mass index, 27-40) nondiabetic, premenopausal women. (my highlights)

Intervention:

Participants were randomly assigned to follow the Atkins (n = 77), Zone (n = 79), LEARN (n = 79), or Ornish (n = 76) diets and received weekly instruction for two months then an additional ten-month follow-up.

Main Outcome Measure:

Weight loss at twelve months was the primary outcome. Secondary outcomes included lipid profile (low-density lipoprotein, high-density lipoprotein, and nonhigh-density lipoprotein cholesterol and triglyceride levels), percentage of body fat, waist-hip ratio, fasting insulin and glucose levels, and blood pressure. Outcomes were assessed at months 0, 2, 6, and 12. The Tukey studentized range test was used to adjust for multiple testing.

Results:

Weight loss was greater for women in the Atkins diet group compared with the other diet groups at twelve months, and mean twelve-month weight loss was significantly different between the Atkins and Zone diets (P < 0.05). Mean twelve-month weight loss was as follows: Atkins, −4.7 kg (95% confidence interval [CI], −6.3 kg to −3.1 kg), Zone, −1.6 kg (95% CI, −2.8 kg to −0.4 kg), LEARN, −2.6 kg (−3.8 kg to −1.3 kg), and Ornish, −2.2 kg (−3.6 kg to −0.8 kg). The weight loss was not statistically different among the Zone, LEARN, and Ornish groups. At twelve months, secondary outcomes for the Atkins group were comparable with or more favorable than the other diet groups.

Conclusions:

In this study, premenopausal overweight and obese women assigned to follow the Atkins diet, which had the lowest carbohydrate intake, lost more weight at twelve months than women assigned to follow the Zone diet and had experienced comparable or more favorable metabolic effects than those assigned to the Zone, Ornish, or LEARN diets [corrected]. While questions remain about long-term effects and mechanisms, a low-carbohydrate, high-protein, high-fat diet may be considered a feasible alternative recommendation for weight loss. (author's highlight)

On page 970 of the A-Z trial, it states, "The Atkins group aimed for 20 g/d or less of carbohydrate for 'induction' (usually 2-3 months) and 50 g/d or less of carbohydrate for the subsequent 'ongoing weight loss' phase."

Sachs Trial

Sachs trial in *NEJM* in February 2009 had 811 participants with 645 participants completing the trial at the end of twenty-four months. That's a dropout rate of 20%.

N Engl J Med. 2009 Feb 26; 360(9):859-73.
Comparison of Weight-Loss Diets with Different Compositions of Fat, Protein, and Carbohydrates. Sachs FM, Bray GA, Carey VJ, Smith SR, Ryan DH, Anton SD, McManus K, Champagne CM, Bishop LM, Laranjo N, Leboff MS, Rood JC, de Jonge L, Greenway FL, Loria CM, Obarzanek E, and Williamson DA.
Source: Department of Nutrition, Harvard School of Public Health, Boston, USA.

Abstract

Background:

The possible advantage for weight loss of a diet that emphasizes protein, fat, or carbohydrates has not been established, and there are few studies that extend beyond one year.

Methods:

We randomly assigned 811 overweight adults to one of four diets; the targeted percentages of energy derived from fat, protein, and carbohydrates in the four diets were 20%, 15%, and 65%; 20%, 25%, and 55%; 40%, 15%, and 45%; and 40%, 25%, and 35%. The diets consisted of similar foods and met guidelines for cardiovascular health. The participants were offered group and individual instructional sessions for two years. The primary outcome was the change in body weight after two years in two-by-two factorial comparisons of low fat versus high fat and average protein versus high protein and in the comparison of highest and lowest carbohydrate content.

Results:

At six months, participants assigned to each diet had lost an average of 6 kg, which represented 7% of their initial weight; they began to regain weight after twelve months. By two years, weight loss remained similar in those who were assigned to a diet with 15% protein and those assigned to a diet with 25% protein (3.0 kg and 3.6 kg, respectively); in those assigned to a diet with 20% fat and those assigned to a diet with 40% fat (3.3 kg for both groups); and in those assigned to a diet with 65% carbohydrates and those assigned to a diet with 35% carbohydrates (2.9 kg and 3.4 kg, respectively) ($P > 0.20$ for all comparisons). Among the 80% of participants who completed the trial, the average weight loss was 4 kg; 14-15% of the participants had a reduction of at least 10% of their initial body weight. Satiety, hunger, satisfaction with the diet, and attendance at group sessions were similar for all diets; attendance was strongly associated with weight loss (0.2 kg per session attended). The diets improved lipid-related risk factors and fasting insulin levels.

Conclusion:

Reduced-calorie diets result in clinically meaningful weight loss regardless of which macronutrients they emphasize. (my highlight: ClinicalTrials.gov number, NCT00072995.)

2009 Massachusetts Medical Society

Comment in
Curr Diab Rep. 2010 Jun; 10(3):165-9.

On page 863, table 1 states the high-fat, high-protein dieters ate 1979 +/— 599 calories in 102 of the 201 participants in the Atkins-style diet. Thirty-five percent of 2,000 calories is 700 calories from carbohydrates: 700 / 4 = 175 g/d of carbohydrates. This is very far from the induction phase advised by Atkins of less than 20 g/d of carbs. Twenty grams of carbohydrate is 80 calories. There are 4 calories for each gram of carbohydrate.

The A-Z trial kept the carbs to 20 g/d for two to three months and then 50 g/d.

50 × 4 = 200 calories.

Tubby Thought

Metabolism

Ancel Keys: Metabolism slowed 40% lower than before study started. p. 109. *Rethinking Thin*

Jules Hirsch: Formally fat people burning as much as 24% fewer calories per square meter of their surface area than the calories used by those who were naturally thin. p. 115. *Rethinking Thin.*

Ethan Sims: When thin men got fat, their metabolism increased by 50%. p. 118. *Rethinking Thin.*

Michael Rosenbaum and Rudolph Leibel found that people who lost about 10% of their weight, reduced the amount of calories burned during movement by 42%. p. 113, *The Skinny: On Losing Weight.*

The science of weight loss is wrong. It is not simply the math of calories in and calories out. The metabolic plateau occurs and the weight loss with the low-calorie diet stops. Ancel Keys had men of normal weight go on a weight loss diet. Their metabolism slowed by 40%. They became fixated on food. They acted like people from the WWII concentration camps. Jules Hirsch found the obese had numerous and huge fat cells. People who lost 100 lbs. looked like someone who was never fat, but they were different. By every measurement they seemed liked people who were starving. There were a few people in Dr. Hirsch's group that maintained their weight loss by maintaining themselves in a state of semistarvation. Ethan Sims did a study to get college students to gain weight. He failed. He then used prisoners of normal weight to force them to gain weight. He succeeded. It took four to six months and up to 10,000 calories a day to get them to gain 25 lbs. The prisoners' metabolism increased by 50%. The prisoners' fat cells grew larger but not more in number. After the study, the prisoners had no trouble losing the weight.

Caveat emptor:

This issue about jumping energy expenditure levels is critical. It has much to do about changing the leptin threshold. Thus, in the future, at least two drugs will be needed. One to lose weight and one to keep the leptin threshold at a point that will not slow our metabolism.

Chapter 23

The Look-AHEAD Trial

"The Look AHEAD trial examined an intensive program in patients who already had diabetes. After one year . . . weight loss . . . was 8.6%. The Look AHEAD trial had included meal replacements that may have accounted for their superior weight loss (compared to 7.5% in the Diabetes Prevention Program)" (Bray, *A Guide to Obesity and the Metabolic Syndrome*, p. 191).

"Wadden et al. 2009 showed a clear effect of adherence to the program on the amount of weight loss achieved. The more sessions people came to, the more weight they lost" (analysis of one-year data; Bray, *A Guide to Obesity and the Metabolic Syndrome*, p. 167).

On the graphs of the article, the four-year data show that despite the intense ongoing behavioral training, the participants decreased exercise and slowly began gaining their weight back.

Tubby Thought

Genetics Is the Gun, Behavior Is the Trigger?

Etiology of Obesity: "Until recently, obesity was considered to be the direct result of a sedentary lifestyle plus chronic ingestion of excess calories. Although these factors are undoubtedly the principal cause in many cases, there is evidence for strong genetic influences on the development of obesity. Adopted children demonstrate a close relationship between their BMI and that of their biologic parents. No such relationship is found between the children and their adoptive parents. Twin studies also demonstrate substantial genetic influences on BMI with little influence from the childhood environment. As much as 40-70% of obesity may be explained by genetic influences."

From: McPhee, Stephen J., Maxine Papdakis, and Michael W. Rabow. *Current Medical Diagnosis and Treatment.* McGraw Hill, 2012.

Caveat emptor:

"Genetics is the gun and behavior the trigger" is the core of the moral hazard argument. The individual is responsible for their obesity. The ignorance of the present state of the science of obesity makes this statement irresponsible.

The Sponge Syndrome explains why genetics trumps behavior in the reduced obese.

Chapter 24

Calories In, Calories Out?

Reasons It's Not Just Calories In and Calories Out as per the First Law of Thermodynamics

1. "To maintain caloric requirements a 62 kg never-obese person requires 1,341 kcal/m2/d, an obese patient requires 1,432 kcal/m2/d.

    The above is not statistically different although, in absolute terms, the obese ate more because of their larger surface areas. A reduced obese person at 100 kg, still obese, requires 1,050 kcal/m2/d."

    From: Liebel RL, Hirsch J. Diminished Energy Requirements-Obese Patients. Metabolism 1984; 33, 164-70.

    This was a study of twenty-six obese patients with an average weight of 152.5 kg. They were hospitalized and fed in a medical ward. This decreased energy expenditure continued for one to two years after weight loss.

2. There is a controversy as to whether it makes a difference if you get high-glycemic carbohydrates or low-glycemic carbohydrates, the latest evidence points to it not making a difference. However, if at some point there is evidence for this, I think it is another example that a calorie is not a calorie. Perhaps if the future

studies compare insulin-resistant patients with noninsulin-resistant obese patients, there will be a difference.

Sichieri R et al., An 18 Mo Randomized Trial of a Low-Glycemic-Index Diet and Weight Change in Brazilian Women. Am J Clin Nutr. 2007; 86(30): 707-13

3.   Ten percent of the population does not respond to exercise.

"Bouchard's group has no immediate plans to reveal to its test participants what their genes reveal about their ability to exercise. But, he says, he knows from all the work so far that some people, about 10% of the population really never get any better with exercise, their endurance will never improve, they will never get faster, and they will never get stronger . . . They did not lose a gram of fat" (Gina Kolata, *Ultimate Fitness* [2003], p. 103).

4.   "Ten % of the population respond astoundingly well" to exercise (*Ultimate Fitness* by Kolata).

5.   As much as 40-70% of obesity may be explained by genetic influences.

"Mutations in MC4R represent the most common genetic cause of severe obesity accounting for 2.5% of all cases. Patients who carry such mutations do not have specific clinical or biological characteristics that differentiate them from other patients with severe obesity; genetic testing is the only reliable method to identify these patients. At present, such testing is not recommended since the presence or absence of one of these mutations carries no specific implications for the clinical management of these patients" (Harrison's 18th edition, *Internal Medicine Text*, 2012).

6.   Metabolism during exercise reduces by 42% after 10% weight loss.

"When my renowned colleagues at Columbia, Dr. Michael Rosenbaum and Dr. Rudolph Leibel, studied the metabolic rates of people who had recently lost 10 per cent of their weight by dieting, they determined this small weight loss slowed calorie burning significant . . . The net reduction was a 42% reduction in the number of calories burned during movement! Whereas most people burn 100 calories for mile they walk, these dieters were burning only 58" (Louis J. Aronne, *The Skinny: On Losing Weight* [2009], p. 112)

7.   After lap band, it takes a week to get to normal metabolic parameters, after Roux en Y, it takes a day. After purely restrictive surgeries, ghrelin levels increase, which may help explain the more dramatic weight loss observed

following RYGB versus purely restrictive surgeries. PYY levels rise to those of a nonobese person following vertical banded gastroplasty. However, with RYGB, there is an early exaggerated response in PYY secretion, approximately two–to fourfold greater than that observed in lean, obese, or gastric banded patients, which may contribute to the sustained weight loss seen with this type of procedure.

Defining appropriate patient criteria to minimize risks and maximize the benefits from bariatric surgery has been debated. Some studies have concluded that surgical intervention is more effective for weight loss and control of comorbid diseases than nonsurgical treatments in patients.

8. Leptin resistance in obese patients.

    It is hypothesized that it is not so much resistance as a threshold below which decreased leptin will cause hunger and reduced metabolic rate and anabolism of fat. The never-obese will reach a very low level of leptin when they lose weight, which will cause them to be hungry, reduce their metabolism, and cause anabolism of fat.

    The reduced obese will reach their leptin threshold at a higher level. This is when they hit the plateau and have difficulty losing any weight. Fat cells make leptin. Fat people have high levels of leptin. This is why giving leptin to fat people does not cause weight loss.

9. Low-carb diet works by using gluconeogenesis, which burns more calories.

10. The Kenyans could not gain enough weight during WWII to qualify to enter the British Army.

11. Patients with insulin resistance have high levels of insulin, which changes the carbs to central obesity quickly and will cause intense hunger, and the carbs are cleared quickly, and the body will not use the fats for energy.

12. Intestinal biodome

    http://www.ncbi.nlm.nih.gov/pubmed/19901833

    Summary:
    Large-scale alterations of the gut microbiota and its microbiome (gene content) are associated with obesity and are responsive to weight loss. Gut microbes can impact host metabolism via signaling pathways in the gut, with

effects on inflammation, insulin resistance, and deposition of energy in fat stores. Restoration of the gut microbiota to a healthy state may ameliorate the conditions associated with obesity and help maintain a healthy weight.

13. Regulation of food intake and energy expenditure

"Obesity is an increase of energy stored as fat that occurs when caloric intake exceeds caloric expenditure. What causes this imbalance is less clear, but recent advances in our understanding of the physiological systems responsible for the maintenance of energy stores in response to variable access to nutrition and demands for energy expenditure have provided some insights into the pathophysiology of obesity. The physiological system controlling food intake and energy expenditure is composed of (1) long-term and short-term afferent signals that allow for sensing the energy status of the individual; (2) integrating brain centers, most importantly within the hypothalamus, where the level of the efferent response is determined; and (3) efferent signals including those regulating the intensity of hunger and the level of energy expenditure.
One common misconception is that this physiological system is dedicated to the prevention of obesity. Instead this system's essential role is in the prevention of starvation (i.e., ensuring adequate energy intake to compensate for the energy requirements of basal metabolism, physical activity, growth, and reproduction). As a result, this physiological system is more strongly biased toward prevention of energy deficiency rather than excess storage."

From: Greenspan's *Basic and Clinical Endocrinology*, 9th edition. McGraw Hill, 2011.

Etiology:
Until recently, obesity was considered to be the direct result of a sedentary lifestyle plus chronic ingestion of excess calories. Although these factors are undoubtedly the principal cause in many cases, there is evidence for strong genetic influences on the development of obesity. Adopted children demonstrate a close relationship between their BMI and that of their biologic parents. No such relationship is found between the children and their adoptive parents. Twin studies also demonstrate substantial genetic influences on BMI with little influence from the childhood environment. As much as 40-70% of obesity may be explained by genetic influences.

Genetic determinants of some types of obesity have now been established. Five genes affecting control of appetite have been identified in mice. Mutations of each gene result in obesity and each has a human homolog. One gene codes for a protein expressed by adipose tissue—leptin—and another for the leptin receptor in the brain. The other three genes affect brain pathways downstream from the leptin receptor. Numerous other candidate genes for human obesity have been identified. Only a small percentage (4-6%) of human obesity is thought to be due to single gene mutations. Most human obesity undoubtedly develops from the interactions of multiple genes, environmental factors, and behavior. The rapid increase in obesity in the last several decades clearly points to a major role of environmental factors in the development of obesity.

McPhee, Stephen J., Maxine Papdakis, and Michael W. Rabow. *Current Medical Diagnosis and Treatment.* McGraw Hill, 2012.

Biology of Obesity: Introduction
In a world where food supplies are intermittent, the ability to store energy in excess of what is required for immediate use is essential for survival. Fat cells, residing within widely distributed adipose tissue depots, are adapted to store excess energy efficiently as triglyceride and, when needed, to release stored energy as free fatty acids for use at other sites. This physiologic system, orchestrated through endocrine and neural pathways, permits humans to survive starvation for as long as several months. However, in the presence of nutritional abundance and a sedentary lifestyle and influenced importantly by genetic endowment, this system increases adipose energy stores and produces adverse health consequences.

From: Longo, Fauci, Kasper, Hauser, Jameson, and Loscalzo. *Harrison's Principles of Internal Medicine.* 18th edition. McGraw Hill, 2012.

14. *Conclusions*
Abdominal visceral fat accumulation, blood pressure, and lipid profile were significantly associated with serum chemerin levels. Our findings suggest that chemerin may be a mediator that links visceral obesity to cardiovascular risk factors.

15. After losing weight, the fat cells don't disappear—they shrink. These cells are ready for fat accumulation as soon as the tubby has a momentary lapse spurred on by a hunger the Twiggies never experience.

Tubby Thought

Antioxidants

Epidemiological and clinical trial evidence surrounding the benefit of B vitamins and antioxidants such as carotenoids, vitamin E, and vitamin C have been contradictory. While pharmacological supplementation of these vitamins in populations with existing CHD has been ineffective and, in some cases, even detrimental, data repeatedly show that consumption of a healthy dietary pattern has considerable cardioprotective effects for primary prevention. Coronary heart disease prevention: nutrients, foods, and dietary patterns.
Bhupathiraju SN, Tucker KL.

From;
Coronary heart disease prevention: nutrients, foods, and dietary patterns.
Bhupathiraju SN, Tucker KL.

Chapter 25

Healthy Diet

Eat healthy!

This is what I hear on TV all the time.

Fruits, vegetables in a variety of colors, nuts, grains, low fats. Low glycemic carbs and plenty of exercise. Portion control, of course. Eat slow. Sit down to eat. Eat breakfast. Chew your food twenty-four times before you swallow it. Take a multivitamin. Take high doses of vitamin D and calcium citrate. Eat fiber. Eat natural or real food, not processed food. Best of all, if you can do it, avoid all animal fats and become a vegetarian. Decrease your calorie intake by 500 calories a day. Weigh yourself every day.

If the above program worked, there would be more weight loss programs that maintained weight loss for five years. Right now that is still about 5%.

Behavior is not the key. Absolute number of calories is not the key. Fat versus carbohydrates is not the key. Most of our fruits, vegetables, and meats are genetically engineered. The corn that organic farmers grow is not the natural corn the Aztecs ate. The Southeast Asians (Indian Hindus) in the USA are dying early on their vegetarian diet probably due to excess carbohydrates causing the metabolic syndrome.

BRIAN S. EDWARDS MD

My biggest objection is about eating for antioxidants. To my knowledge, there is no outcome data for this. There has been data that vitamins A, C, and E have no special advantage in high doses. The Lyon trial is often touted as an example of a healthy diet in what we call the Mediterranean diet. There are many confounding covariables in this trial. Lately, it's not the olive oil that is the special ingredient. It is a whole lifestyle that made the diet "healthy."

Genetics and physiology are the key. Perhaps the tubby genetics is designed to survive the next ice age. Presently food is plentiful. Carbohydrates in particular are cheap and taste good and generate hunger in three hours due to insulin surge. No more manufacturing or farming; sedentary lifestyle with TV and computers. This has thrown our nation into large waists and the metabolic syndrome. The new adipocytes produce leptin. Some say we become leptin resistant; others say the leptin threshold is very high in the obese.

Going from thin to tubby with the metabolic syndrome has made Tubbies insulin resistant. This is the beginning of a new physiology that makes it very difficult to go back to normal physiology. I believe that when Senator McGovern told us to eat a low-fat, high-carb diet, he did a great disservice to the country. It coincided with the obesity epidemic. The ADA changed its 40-40-20 diet to a low-fat, high-carb diet with little evidence to back up the change. There was a real concern that high-fat diet will cause higher cholesterol and more cardiovascular deaths. I am on a 60% fat diet, and I have shown that for my tubby metabolism on Crestor 5 mg and Niacin 1,000 mg, my LDL-P has not gone up after one year. The A-Z trial and the Sachs comparative diet trial have shown high-fat diet to be lipid neutral. The recent meta-analysis has shown that high-saturated-fat diets are no worse than low-fat diets. The dieticians tell me this is only true with weight loss. I demonstrated after a year of 60% fat and no weight loss a good lipid profile. Remember on a cruise, when you fill your plate with ten types of colorful fruit, it is not healthy if you have metabolic syndrome. Most people with big waists are insulin resistant. Get rid of the carbohydrates and don't worry about the antioxidants. Peroxide permutase is 100,00 times stronger than the antioxidant in blueberries. Your body makes peroxide permutase, and it increases with exercise.

From the title page below:
"Epidemiological and clinical trial evidence surrounding the benefit of B vitamins and antioxidants such as carotenoids, vitamin E, and vitamin C, have been contradictory. While pharmacological supplementation of these vitamins in populations with existing CHD has been ineffective and, in some cases, even detrimental, data repeatedly show that consumption of a healthy dietary pattern has considerable cardioprotective effects for primary prevention."

"The strongest and most consistent protective associations are seen with fruit and vegetables, fish, and whole grains."

I just do not believe this is true for the reduced obese with metabolic syndrome. I don't think the studies have been done on this subset.

"Several epidemiological studies show that people following the Mediterranean style diet or the Dietary Approaches to Stop Hypertension (DASH) diet have lower risk of CHD and lower likelihood of developing hypertension."

The DASH diet is low in salt. Good for people who have salt-sensitive hypertension.
The Mediterranean diet is very nebulous. The Lyon study may have more to do with lifestyle. Olive oil is hotly debated as the key ingredient. It is a 55% fat diet, I believe.

I am willing to agree that DASH and the Lyon diet and lifestyle have been shown to be healthy diets in certain population groups. However, "evidence on changes in dietary patterns and changes in CHD risk is still emerging."

I believe that people with metabolic syndrome or insulin resistance do poorly with diets that replace low fat with carbohydrates.

I also believe that starving teenagers to lose weight sets them up for morbid obesity later in life. It messes up with their metabolism. Low-calorie diets fail. They are not sustainable. Our kids should eat butter, animal fat, and whole milk. It will satiate them so they don't snack on carbohydrates. Vegan diets are, by nature, high carbohydrate. The South Asian Indians are vegetarians. The carbohydrates they eat in the States are killing them with their metabolic syndrome.

Tubby Thought

Cholesterol Threshold

Cholesterol threshold: After 300 mg of cholesterol in your diet, it doesn't matter much how much cholesterol you have in your diet. It does not increase your risk much. More than half the calories found in eggs come from the fat in the yolk; a large (50 g) chicken egg contains approximately 5 g of fat.

Cholesterol does not contain calories.

Most of the risk of Cholesterol consumption comes from the first 200 mg ingested. It is very difficult to have a diet with no cholesterol.

The liver makes most of the cholesterol in the body. Your cholesterol level is mostly dependent on your genetics rather than the amount of cholesterol you eat.

Rather than worry about the amount of cholesterol in your food, get your blood level of LDL-P to less than 750 with statins and niacin.

Chapter 26

How Does a Low-Carbohydrate Diet Work?

"Several mechanism have been suggested for the possible added value of Low Carbohydrate diets in promoting weight loss, including

1. higher amounts of protein (which produces satiety more than carbohydrates)
2. ongoing gluconeogenesis to compensate for the body's carbohydrate needs, which is an energy-consuming process.
3. increased diuresis
4. loss of glycogen stores and their associated water.
5. high levels of circulating ketones, which suppresses appetite.
6. limited food choices
7. under reporting of food intake by the LC (low carbohydrate) group"

This list is from Medical Clinic of North America. Obesity. p. 943. Authors: Dubnov-Raz and Berry.

It is often said that very low-carbohydrate diets provide lower total calories for the day. When I order a hamburger for lunch, I put the bun and French fries on a separate plate. If I had eaten those carbs, I would have been hungry again in two to three hours. Instead, I have a larger burger with cheese and bacon. I may eat less calories on my low-carb diet compared to my old diet when I ate everything on my plate.

As one reads the medical literature, especially the meta-analysis, one must be very careful to realize most of the studies were done with a small number of people for a short time.

The three most important studies that are random controlled head to head:

Gardner CD et al., JAMA 2007; 297(9): 969-77. A-Z trial.
311 overweight women; 260 premenopausal women finished the diet. It lasted one year.
20% attrition rate
12-month trial
The Atkins produced more weight loss at six and twelve months.

Shai I. et al., N Engl J Med 2008; 359:229-41.
322 overweight employees
15% attrition rate
24-month trial
The low-fat diet produced less weight loss.

Sachs's comparison of four diets. NEJMed. 2009
This may be the biggest trial of comparing LC versus LF. It has, unfortunately, by the end of the study, the differences of the macronutrients creep closely together. However, Dr. Bray writes on page 191 in his text that this is the most clear cut of the trials. It had 811 patients and lasted two years, 20% attrition rate. There was no difference in outcome between the four diets; people who adhered to their diet lost the most weight.

Safety issues:

Review of 100 studies identified no adverse effects or unwarranted metabolic changes, especially renal function in the low-carbohydrate diets.
Bravata DM et al. Efficacy and Safety of Low Carbohydrate diets: A Systemic Review. JAMA 2003, 289(14):1837

The body can't store protein. The excess protein is broken down and excreted as nitrogen in ammonia. There is concern about the long-term safety of this on the kidneys and liver. So far, in the Bravata review, this has not been a problem. On page 189 in Dr. Bray's text, "When carbohydrate intake is less than 50 g per day, ketosis uniformly develops. One concern with ketosis is the source of the cations needed to excrete the ketones. If the cations consist of calcium from the bone, this process may enhance the risk of bone loss."

Tubby Thought

Less Than Magic Drugs to Lose Weight

"Scientists have developed a new drug that attacks excess body fat, and a new study reports that it helped a small group of obese monkeys lose weight. But researchers at the M. D. Anderson Cancer Center in Houston designed the new drug Adipotide to attack the fat itself by destroying the blood supply that keeps it alive. "Without the blood supply, the fat withers away and is re-metabolized by the liver," said Dr. Wadih Arap, one of the study's authors.

Four weeks after the monkeys stopped taking the drug, they began to regain their weight. Dr. Keith Ayoob, associate professor in pediatrics in the Albert Einstein College of Medicine in Bronx, NY, said that fact makes the drug like many of its less-than-magical predecessors.

"We've always been able to get people to lose weight, but the real question is how to keep the lost weight from returning. Right now, there's no drug for that," Ayoob said. By Carrie Gann (@carrie_gann), ABC News Medical Unit, Nov. 9, 2011.

Caveat emptor:

Fen-phen was a great drug combination to lose weight, but when twenty million people took it and took it in large doses, there were problems with it.

Instead of embracing bariatric surgery we need to accept drugs with black box warnings and use them cautiously in the way we learned to use statins correctly. Unfortunately, we have not found the magic drug to change the leptin threshold or prevent the plateau or the resettlement point or whatever we end up calling it.

Chapter 27

Victoza (Liraglutide) May Be the New Miracle Drug

There are endocrine changes after bariatric surgery bypassing the foregut or midgut from feeding. Roux-en-Y gastric bypass.

"Incretins are gastrointestinal hormones that directly stimulate insulin release from Beta cells of the pancreas, and whose reduced secretion is theorized to significantly contribute to type 2 diabetes."

"Endogenous GLP-1 (glucagon-like peptide 1) is made by L cells of the colon and ileum. Mechanisms of action include:

1. direct stimulation of insulin secretion
2. inhibition of glucagon secretion
3. augmentation of the Beta cell mass
4. delayed gastric emptying and acid production
5. increase satiety

Levels (of GLP-1) increase after carbohydrate intake and have been shown to increase in a non-statistical significant way after gastric bypass." p.1024

Smith et al.
Surgical Approaches to the Treatment of Obesity
Obesity Medical Clinics of North America
September 2011, volume 95, number 5

Actos is known to increase peripheral weight while decreasing glucose. Victoza or liraglutide (a 3.0 mg daily injectable) is a GLP-1 agonist that has a 97% homology to GLP-1 and may be a good substitute for Actos in type 2 diabetics. Liraglutide has shown to produce weight loss but does not have that indication yet.

Caveat emptor:

I took Victoza injections 0.6 mg for twelve days starting on 12-31-11. Victoza caused me to have an upset stomach, decreased appetite, and decreased desire for alcohol. On the thirteenth day, the side effects seemed less. I increased my Victoza dose to 1.2 mg. The side effects returned. I did not eat large portions as I was told that might cause vomiting. After a month of Victoza I lost approximately 10 lbs. while staying on 40 g of carbs a day. My appetite remains less but no more sick stomach and I enjoy my food again. I started Victoza injections about a week before I went on my World Cruise. The side effects were significant. Chemotherapy for cancer often have severe side effects. I was willing to suffer the side effects in order to get my fasting glucose down. My fasting glucose has improved from 230 to 150. I am walking ninety minutes a day on the deck. Byetta injections are available as once a week shots. I have no experience with the weekly dose.

Tubby Thought

Even Physics Has Controversy

Bell's theorem has great importance for physics and the philosophy of science, as it implies that quantum physics must necessarily violate either the principle of locality or counterfactual definiteness.[1] It is the most famous legacy of the Irish mathematician, John Stewart Bell.

Caveat emptor:

Even in the hard world of physics, there is continued controversy as to whether Einstein or Born was right about quantum mechanics. The Irish mathematician John Steward Bell recently added some weight to Einstein's side about quantum mechanics. Dr. Bell had a difficult time finding an experimental physicist to test Dr. Bell's theorem. It took a younger physicist to do the experiment. The eminent professors felt it was a waste of time. All I am saying is we need more humility when making declarative statements in a science as fuzzy as nutrition. Let's not tell the country this is a healthy diet when we really don't know.

"Matrices: Arrays of numbers (or other elements such as variables) with their own rules of algebra, matrices are extremely useful for expressing information about a physical system.
An nxn square matrix has n columns and n rows."

"Heisenberg's ignorance of the accepted rules and regulations of quantum physics allowed him to tread where others, welded to a more cautious and rational approach, feared to."

"His (Heisenberg) new physics appeared to work only with the help of a strange kind of multiplication, where X times Y did not equal Y times X. With ordinary numbers it did not matter in which order they were multiplied: 4 × 5 gives exactly the same answer as 5 × 4, 20. Mathematicians called this property, where the ordering in multiplication is unimportant, commutation. Numbers obey the commutative law of multiplication, so (4 × 5) − (5 × 4) is always zero . . . Heisenberg was deeply troubled by the discovery that when he multiplied two arrays together, the answer was dependent on the order in which they were multiplied. (AXB) − (BXA) was not always zero."

Quotes are from *Quantum, Einstein, Bohr, and the Great Debate about the Nature of Reality* by Manjit Kumar.

Chapter 28

Cancer Update

This is a government report. The decrease in cancer is not from eating blueberries. It is from screening for cancer and medical treatment. Stopping smoking has decreased the deaths from cancer. We still are not clear what role fat and carbs have on cancer. Recently a Swedish study found processed meat to be unhealthy. My point is that fruits and vegetables are not the cure they are all made out to be, especially with tubby patients with insulin resistance.

Other highlights of the reports:

Cancer kills Americans at the rate of about 1,500 people a day.

Lung cancer accounts for more deaths than any other cancer among both men and women.

The probability of being diagnosed with an invasive cancer during your life is 44% for men and 38% for women.

For men, prostate, lung and bronchus (respiratory system tissue), and colon cancer account for about 52% of all newly diagnosed cancers. Prostate cancer accounts for 29% of cases in men.

The three most common types of cancer in women in 2011 are breast, lung and bronchus, and colon, which, when combined, account for about 53% of cancer cases in women. Breast cancer alone accounts for 30% of the cases.

Lung and bronchus, breast, and colon combined account for almost 50% of cancer deaths among men and women.

Declines in colon cancer deaths reflect increased screening for the disease.

For men, the reduction in deaths from lung, prostate, and colon cancer make up about 80% of the total decrease in the cancer deaths.

For women, a decline in deaths from breast and colon cancers accounts for about 60% of the decrease.

This year, the American Cancer Society expects 1,596,670 new cancer cases and 571,950 deaths from the disease in the United States.

By Steve Sternberg, USA TODAY
http://www.usatoday.com/community/tags/reporter.aspx?id=594

Heart disease deaths in the USA have fallen below the American Heart Association's prevention goal for 2010, and deaths from strokes are nearing their own record low, the AHA said Tuesday.

But epidemics of diabetes, obesity, and inactivity, along with widespread racial, economic, and geographic differences in access to care, threaten those gains, warns AHA president Daniel Jones.

"Unless we can find a new strategy to stem diabetes and obesity, we can anticipate a new wave of cardiovascular disease deaths," Jones says. He noted that heart disease is still the nation's leading killer, and stroke ranks third.

New government data show that heart disease death rates dropped 25.8%, between 1999 and 2005, from 195 to 144 deaths for every 100,000 people, surpassing the AHA's 25% target reduction. Stroke deaths dropped 24.4%, from sixty-one to forty-seven deaths per 100,000.

That adds up to roughly 160,000 lives saved in 2005, Jones says. If the trend holds, the AHA projects that as many as 240,000 lives may be saved this year.

The analysis of data released by the National Center for Health Statistics doesn't explain why death rates continue to fall. Studies suggest people are eating better, smoking less and getting better medical care than Americans of previous generations, says Paul Ridker of Brigham and Women's Hospital in Boston.

Ridker says improved methods of preventing and treating cardiovascular disease have paid off. "Not only have they reduced the number of events, but when events occur, we're more likely to survive them," he says.

These advances didn't benefit everyone, AHA notes. The death rate for blacks dropped by 23.8%, compared with 25.6% for whites. "While overall statistics look better for the U.S. as a whole," Ridker says, "a major portion of our population is not benefiting from this shift."

Heart disease death rates fell among women by 26.9%, and stroke deaths among women were down 23.7%.

Signs of trouble loom on the horizon, among them twin epidemics of diabetes and obesity in young people, says Daniel Levy of the National Heart, Lung, and Blood Institute's Framingham study, a fifty-year-old examination of heart disease in a Massachusetts community.

"We haven't yet paid the full price in heart disease and stroke deaths for the obesity epidemic in our children that began 25 years ago," he says.

I believe if we screen for plaque with CIMT and CAC early in people with at least one risk factor and then treat with statin and Endur-acin to a LDL-P goal of < 750, we will prevent most cardiovascular deaths. Assuming the patients have controlled their hypertension and stopped smoking. We need to focus on the tubby approach as opposed to diet and exercise.

The Bari 2D and the Courage trial show that medicine is as good as stents and surgery in late coronary disease. I propose we start treating earlier than that. We need preventive medicine that is inexpensive and safe. Simvastatin and Endur-acin cost $100 a year. We can screen for disease with CIMT and CAC for $150.

From Harrison's *Principles of Internal Medicine*, 18th edition, 2012, McGraw Hill, p. 655:
"International epidemiologic studies suggest that diets high in fat are associated with increased risk for cancers of the breast, colon, prostate and endometrium . . . Despite correlations, dietary fat has not been proven to cause cancer." p. 656: "Two large prospective cohort studies of > 100,000 health professionals showed no association between fruit and vegetable intake and risk of cancer."

"The U.S. National Institutes of Health Women's Health Initiative launched in 1994, was a long term clinical trial enrolling > 100,000 women aged 45-69 years. It placed women in 22 intervention groups . . . The study showed that while dietary fat intake was lower in the diet intervention group, invasive breast cancers were not reduced over an 8-year follow-up period compared to the control group. No reduction was seen in the incidence of colorectal cancer in the dietary intervention arm. The difference in dietary fat averaged ~10% between the two groups. Evidence does not currently establish the anti-carcinogenic value of vitamin, mineral or nutritional supplements in amounts greater than those provided by a balanced diet."

Introduction to Clinical Nutrition. 3rd edition. Vishwanath Sardesai. CRC press. 2012. p. 6:
Red and Processed Meats–Less Is Better

"A second study of nearly 150,000 adults has found that eating too much red and processed meat increases a person's risk of colorectal cancer by up to 50%."
Sinha, R. et al. 2009. Meat Intake and Mortality: A Prospective Study of Over Half a Million People. Arch Intern Med 169562

Nutrition Concepts & Controversies. 2011. Sizer and Whitney. p. 221:
Defense Against Cancer

"In a 2007 report, cancer authorities (American Institute of Cancer Research) made this statement: 'Red meat is a convincing cause of colorectal cancer.'"

"Not so fast" is the answer from a surprising study of over 60,000 people in the United Kingdom. "In this study people who ate fish but not red meats had the lowest overall cancer rates . . . Vegetarians also had lower rates than meat eaters for total cancers . . . However, vegetarians had the highest number of colon and rectal cancers of any group while fish eaters had the lowest rate"
T. J. Key et al., Cancer Incidence in Vegetarians: Results from the European Prospective Investigation into Cancer and Nutrition, *American Journal of Clinical Nutrition,* 89(209): 1620s-1626s.

In Vishwanath's Clinical nutrition book paragraph on eating less meat, he seems to leave out the rest of the story. Mozaffarian states that people who eat less red meat (and choose poultry and fish most often) may also adopt other healthy habits, such as exercising regularly, which may reduce the cancer risk. This added analysis was found in the Sizer and Whitney nutrition text.

R. Shinha et al., Meat Intake and Mortality: A Prospective Study of Over Half a Million People, Archives of Internal Medicine 169(2009): 543-545.
D. Mozaffarian, Higher Red Meat Intake May Be a Marker of Risk, Not a Risk Factor Itself, Archives of Internal Medicine 169(2009): 1538-1539.

Tubby Thought

2001 NCEP: ATP III and IDF Criteria for Metabolic Syndrome:

Waist Circumference:

Men	Women	Ethnicity
> 93 CM	> 79 CM	Europid, sub-Saharan African and Middle Eastern
> 89 CM	> 79 CM	South Asian, ethnic South and Central American
> 84 CM	> 89 CM	Japanese

Caveat emptor:

"Measuring waist circumference does not reliably distinguish increases in subcutaneous adipose tissue vs. visceral fat; this distinction requires CT or MRI . . . Relative increases in visceral versus subcutaneous adipose tissue with increasing waist circumference in Asians and Asian Indians may explain the greater prevalence of the syndrome in those populations compared with African-American men in whom subcutaneous fat predominates" (Robert H. Eckel, "Metabolic Syndrome," in Harrison's Principles of Internal Medicine, 18th edition [2012], pp. 1993-1994).

Chapter 29

Twiggies May Also Have Metabolic Syndrome

I am a natural-born tubby. My best friend is a natural-born twiggy. I always wanted to get down to his weight, and he wanted to bulk up a bit. We went to Stuyvesant High School together in Manhattan, NYC. During those years, I would try to follow Weight Watchers diet. He would stop on the way to the subway to get a vanilla malted milk shake. I had given those up. We both exercised with daily basketball or weight lifting. He ran the 600 m one second faster than me. He could dunk a tennis ball; I could touch the rim. We were both 5'11.75".

We went to Brooklyn College together. City college was free back then. We grew up in similar environments and were very athletic. He never worried about what he ate. I had to watch it all the time, and despite vigorous daily basketball, I struggled with my weight, and he did not. We often ate together.

His nature was different from mine. He could not binge on food the way I could. His body didn't want him to. He was always restless. He didn't like watching long movies or watching TV all night. I enjoyed my sedentary moments. I came from the tubby plateau planet, while he came from the twiggy planet.

Now we are fifty-nine. I am diabetic and have a CAC of 8 and CIMT of less than 25%.

He has psoriasis (mild), a CAC of zero, but a CIMT at 70%.

My LDL-P is 750. His LDL-C was 120, with HDL-C of 34 and triglycerides 160. His doctor said he could take some niacin to raise his HDL-C. HDL-C less than 35 is a major risk factor for cardiovascular disease.

I talked him into getting a CAC, CIMT, and LDL-P. His LDL-P was 1,200. He had discordance with LDL-C.

He is not fat. His weight in high school at graduation was 155 lbs., and his waist was

30 inches. In his twenties, he weight was up to 170 lbs. His weight at fifty-nine years old is 183 lbs., and his waist is 34 inches. He overate for a while to put on bulk. He went up to 190 lbs. He gave up on the high calorie diet and easily went back to 183 lbs.

Does he have metabolic syndrome? He has a triglyceride/HDL disorder. His fasting glucose is normal. He still exercises a lot. He doesn't have a forty-inch waist, but his waist has increased, and if we do a CT of his abdomen, we might find a large amount of central fat. Japanese men have a metabolic syndrome waist of thirty-five inches.

Since he has atherosclerosis as demonstrated by his CIMT of 70%, and he has two major risk factors—age more than forty-five years old and HDL-C less than thirty-five—and an inflammatory disorder called psoriasis, I urged him to take statin and Endur-acin to reverse plaque buildup and to follow his CIMT every two to three years. His primary physician was angry with me for interfering.

His liposcience panel:	8-10	10-26-10	6-2011
LDL-P	1212	792	724

He responded well to Simvastatin and Endur-acin as demonstrated in the later two lab results above.

Consult 10-2010:

The patient is a fifty-nine-year-old man with a history of psoriasis. This inflammatory disorder can put him at increased risk for atherosclerosis. The lipid panel is a classic example of discordance with the traditional LDL-C and the new method of NMR LDL-particle number. The patient believed that his "cholesterol" was good because his LDL-C runs around 100. It was 100 on this test before medication. However, the LDL-P was 1,212. At this level, atherosclerosis occurs as per NCEP guidelines.

His CAC or calcium score was zero, and this predicts that it is very unlikely for him to have a cardiac event in the next three years. However, CAC does not rule out coronary atherosclerosis.

Further testing with CIMT proved him to have atherosclerosis with a CIMT around 70%. This means his carotid wall is thicker than 70% of men his age.

Diagnosis:

Atherosclerosis
Atheroma of Carotids
Psoriasis
Possible Metabolic Syndrome (as per the HDL/triglyceride axis disorder)
HDL-P is low at 28
LDL-P is high at 1,212
Triglycerides high at 191 (nonfasting)
Non-HDL cholesterol high at 138

Goal is to get reversal of atheroma of carotids on CIMT in two years:

LDL-P < 750
Non-HDL cholesterol < 80
Triglycerides < 100 fasting
HDL-P > 35

Personally, I think if we get the LDL-P to less than 750, we will not need to worry about the other numbers. The recent AIM HIGH trial supports this notion.

After the above LDL-P test was done, his physician put him on Simvastatin. The patient started taking Endur-acin 500 mg bid with meals. It is now two months after the patient took the lipid lowering medicine, and I have sent in a prescription for a repeat LDL-P. The patient has discordance with his LDL-C. The LDL-C is insufficient to properly follow the response to therapy. If the patients LDL-P is less than 500, we can decrease his Simvastatin in half as that is important to him. However, if the LDL-P goes back to more than 750, I would resume the full initial dose of Simvastatin that he has been taking.

I appreciate the opportunity to contribute to my friend's prevention of heart attack and stroke from the inflammation of psoriasis. My friend has a classic case of subclinical atherosclerosis and discordance of LDL-C.

Thank you,

Brian S. Edwards, MD
Diplomate and Fellow of the National Lipid Association

Tubby Thought

Leptin

"The discovery of leptin catapulted the fat cell into the arena of endocrine cells (Zhang et al.). The finding of a peptide released from fat cells that acts at a distance has refocused interest in the fat cell from primarily a cell that stores fatty acids to a cell with important endocrine and paracrine functions . . . The endocrine products produced and secreted by the fat cell number close to 100
(Halberg, Wenstedt, and Scherer 2009)"
(George Bray, A Guide to Obesity and the Metabolic Syndrome, p. 87).

Chapter 30

Update on the Tubby Theory from Topeka

I don't think I need to write a new edition of my tubby theory. The NCEP has not yet updated their guidelines. The AIM TRIAL showed no benefit in lowering triglycerides and raising HDL-C in patients that already achieved an LDL-C goal of <80 with a statin. This trial ended too soon, and there is a confounding covariable of adding Zetia to the control group.

In my *Tubby Theory* book, I followed what Dr. Dayspring has taught. The LDL-P goal is most important and the size of the LDL-C does not matter either.

I prefer combination therapy with niacin (Endur-acin) as it improves compliance by not subjecting the patient to the highest dose of statin. My exercise advice is basically the same. Walk at least eight minutes a day. Since my book was published I learned that being sedentary for eight hours is very bad. The diet I advised was based on keeping saturated fats done to 7%. I no longer believe that, as this new book attests. Lipitor is now available as its generic form: Atorvastatin. This is a much stronger and safer drug than Simvastatin and I would advise switching patients to Atrovastatin. Zetia is still waiting on its outcome data. I would use Zetia only as a third drug or selected cases as a second drug.

I have been reading Dr. Siddhartha Mukherjee's book *The Emperor of All Maladies: A Biography of Cancer.*

I can strongly recommend this book to everyone. I think the Mary Lasker story can be instructive to us in the National Lipid Association. On pages 231-233, John Bailar and Elaine Smith wrote in the *NEJM*, May 1986, an article about "age adjustment" for mortality analysis in cancer treatment.

"It shook the world of oncology by its roots."

They wrote that "between 1962 and 1985, cancer-related deaths had increased by 8.7%."

"Some thirty-five years of intense effort focused largely on improving treatment must be judged a qualified failure."

"As Cairns had already pointed out, the only intervention ever known to reduce the aggregate mortality for a disease—any disease—at a population level was prevention."

Page 234: "In 1974, describing to Mary Lasker the comprehensive activities of the NCI, the director, Frank Rauscher, wrote effusively about its three-pronged approach to cancer: 'Treatment, Rehabilitation, and Continuing Care.' That there was no mention of either prevention or early detection was symptomatic: the institute did not even consider cancer prevention a core strength."

I am proposing an NLA project to prevent 100,000 sudden coronary deaths each year through the following:

1. Early detection of plaque or atheroma with CAC, CIMT (both independent risk factors in the MESA trial). (Cost for two tests in my area is $150.)
2. Inexpensive combination therapy with generic statin and niacin (OTC brand Endur-acin causes little flushing). (Costs $100 a year.)
3. Goal to reduce LDL-P to less than 750 to regress plaque (or apoB less than 60, I am concerned about reliability of apoB immunoassay in people with metabolic syndrome).
4. Follow up CIMT in three years to determine effectiveness of treatment.

This is inexpensive and safe "secondary prevention" program. Generic Lipitor will be available and is even safer and stronger than generic Zocor. Critical step is to start at low dose of statin to avoid muscle side effects and losing a patient forever to taking statins.

Adding 1,000 mg of niacin decreases LDL-C by 16%. We need a niacin that will allow compliance in a big group. It has been my experience that over-the-counter

Endur-acin at 500 mg bid with meals rarely causes flushing. I take 1,000 mg at a time and experience a mild flush. At 1,000 mg, niacin rarely causes increase in liver function tests or glucose.

Compliance is critical in the success of a large program. Cost is critical. I think Endur-acin is cheaper than Slo-Niacin, and the wax mattress allows the patient to break the tablet in half if tapering up dose is needed. Niaspan is a brand that should be used when doses greater than 1,000 mg are needed because of cost and flushing.

Let's step forward boldly and make a statement of prevention and early treatment.

If a woman tests positive for BRCA-1, she may get prophylactic bilateral mastectomies or start taking Tamoxifen prophylactically for the rest of her life.

In Nature (1993), Druker describes adding CGP57148 to leukemia cells from a human marrow in a petri dish. He cured leukemia in the dish.

Ciba-Geigy did not want to spend $200 million on trials for a drug that would treat CML (chronic myeloid leukemia) as this disease only afflicts only a few thousand people a year.

Druker persisted, and by 1998, he witnessed dozens of remissions in CML with this drug. It was then marketed as Gleevec.

As of 2009, author Siddhartha Mukherjee writes in his book *The Emperor of All Maladies*, on page 440: "As of 2009, CML patients treated with Gleevec survive an average of thirty years after their diagnosis. Based on that survival figure, Hagop Kantarjian estimates that within the next decade, 250,000 people will be living with CML in America, all of them on targeted therapy."

We can diagnose atherosclerosis with a CAC of more than 1 or a CIMT at 1.0 mm or 75% tile.
We can treat plaque for $100 a year with generic statin and OTC niacin.

One hundred thousand people a year die from sudden coronary death. Thirty to 50% die with sudden coronary death as the first symptom. Imagine the number of people alive thirty years from now based on a modest survival figure of 30,000 people a year saved from subclinical atherosclerosis.

Right now we have no program to find these people and treat them. Yet CAC and CIMT are available at a reasonable price. Let's do something!

Chapter 31

Epilogue

This case study has five end points:

1. Weight, no change
2. LDL-P, 750-1,200 (transient elevations)
3. CIMT, no change
4. CAC probably no change as last CAC done while I was in atrial fibrillation.
5. Hemoglobin A1C, elevated due to going off Actos in May

I previously showed regression in my CAC and CIMT in my book *The Tubby Theory from Topeka*.

After twelve months of 60% fat, my CIMT may be the most significant indicator. It showed no real change in plaque. My diabetes had a setback when I stopped my Actos for a few months.

A case study does not prove much. I simply hope to raise questions. Low-fat, low-calorie diets have been touted as the way to diet. I have shown that for myself: I could eat 60% fat, mostly animal fat, and not worsen my lipid profile or increase plaque in my arteries over a year.

I have not lost weight, and I led a lifestyle that had less exercise. I did not count calories. I was not hungry. I drank alcohol. I did not gain weight. I went on ninety days of cruises. I usually gained weight when I did road trips and sat in the car for eight to twelve hours.

For more than three years I exercised two to three hours a day. I continued to gain weight because I had Sponge Syndrome. I stopped eating carbohydrates, especially fruit and bread. My Hgb A1C improved with less exercise. My LDL-C did not get worse. My LDL-P fluctuated a little but often was excellent at 750. I finally stopped the inexorable gain toward my former maximum weight of 280, and I did it with less exercise and not feeling hungry. There is a lot to be said for this. I am not saying low-carbohydrate diet is for everyone, but for people with metabolic syndrome, prediabetes, or diabetes it should be tried. If it is tried, the tubby theory should be incorporated, and LDL-P, CAC, and CIMT should be followed.

I would like to see future studies use the low-carbohydrate diets with metabolic syndrome using the tubby criteria–CIMT, CAC, and LDL-P. It is also important to not concentrate so much on behavioral eating but instead to have improved compliance with continued low carbohydrates.

Another arm of the study needs to be to study those with GG genome and put them on a low-fat diet. There needs to be a sea change informing people of the futility of low-calorie diets because of the Sponge Syndrome.

Physicians need to identify metabolic syndrome patients and teach them to eat a very low-carbohydrate diet not to lose weight but to prevent diabetes. Tubbies should walk twenty to sixty minutes a day not to lose weight but to prevent diabetes and further weight gain.

The goals should be to prevent the following:

1. Prevent laying down more plaque with atherosclerosis by keeping LDL-P at 750
2. Gaining more weight
3. Preventing diabetes type 2

These goals can best be achieved most of the time (depending mostly on genetic make-up) with:

1. a low-carbohydrate diet as there is no hunger
2. walking a minimum of twenty minutes a day

A low-fat diet is not safer or better. A low-calorie diet is doomed to fail due to the carbohydrates causing increased hunger, two to three hours after eating them due to the surge of insulin.

A low-carbohydrate diet is restrictive, but if people concentrate on eating 30 g of protein with each meal three times a day and understand that carbs drive insulin, which drive fat accumulation as well as hunger, hopefully they will be more motivated.

It takes about a month to end much of the carbohydrate craving. Eating carbs seems to cause more carb carving. I try to keep it to 20 g, but I have a morning bagel once in a while. I think people can increase to 40-80 g of carbs depending on their exercise schedule; however, to eat more carbs with more fats is a formula for gaining weight and having a poor lipid profile.

I hope I have taken away some of the fear of eating fats and cholesterol. Prove it to yourself by getting an LDL-P blood test every three months. If your LDL-P is going up, ask your physician to put you on low-dose statin and repeat the LDL-P in a month. Better yet, lets have a real outcome study with 5,000 people. Half of the people eat 40g of carbs a day and the other half eat only10% fat for five years.

Check the LDL-P, CIMT and CAC during the course of the five years. Pending this study, do the experiment on yourself under the care of your personal physician.

Remember, if it tastes good, it probably has fat in it, and with protein, it prevents hunger.

Final Word

April 2, 2012

My endocrinologist started me on Victoza injections on Dec. 31, 2011. It definitely has improved my fasting glucose from 220 to 155. It also prevents me from overeating. On Jan. 6, 2012, I boarded the MS *Amsterdam* of Holland American for a 112-day world cruise. On Victoza, I have lost approximately 12 lbs. as of Feb. 4. I try to walk one to two hours a day. I continue a low-carbohydrate diet.

Follow my progress on my blog;
The Tubby Traveler from Topeka, at *http://meandgin. blogspot.com/*

REGRESSION OF PLAQUE

The more astute reader may have noticed that the lab documents did not include the CIMT numbers I reported on earlier.

I used a control CIMT at KUMC with Dr. Patrick Moriarty.

He uses a Sono Cal IMT scan. The results with this machine are:

	12/17/09	12/9/11
Avg. Mean	0.599 mm	0.563 mm
Avg. Max.	0.741 mm	0.661 mm

I gained around 15 pounds in 2010 by eating a lot of fruit.

I stayed the same weight in 2011 despite eating 60% fat in my diet. Mostly animal fat.

The amazing results suggest I had regression of the atheroma in my carotids.

I attribute this to crestor 5 mg, endur-acin 1,000 mg and Lovaza 4,000 for keeping my LDL-P in the 700 to 1,000 range.

Bibliography

Books

Kolata, Gina. *Rethinking Thin: The New Science of Weight Loss—And the Myths and Realities of Dieting*. Farrar, Straus and Giroux, 2007.

Kolata, Gina. *Ultimate Fitness: The Quest for Truth about Exercise and Health*. Farrar, Straus and Giroux, 2003.

Taubes, Gary. *Why We Get Fat: And What to Do about It*. Alfred A. Knopf, 2011.

Aronne, Louis J., and Alisa Bowman. *The Skinny: On Losing Weight Without Being Hungry*.

Cordain, Loren. *The Paleo Diet*. 2002. Revised edition. John Wiley and Sons, 2011.

Bray, George A. *A Guide to Obesity and the Metabolic Syndrome: Origins and Treatment*. CRC Press, 2011.

LeRotih and Karnielli. "Obesity." Medical Clinics of North America, vol. 95, no 5. September 2011.

Texts

Longo, Fauci, Kasper, Hauser, Jameson, Loscalzo. *Harrison's Principles of Internal Medicine*.
18th edition. McGraw Hill, 2012.

McPhee, Stephen J., Maxine Papdakis, and Michael W. Rabow. *Current Medical Diagnosis and Treatment*. McGraw Hill, 2012.

Gardner, David G., and Dolores Shoback. *Greenspan's Basic and Clinical Endocrinology.* 9th edition. McGraw Hill, 2011.

Sizer, Frances Sienkiewicz, and Eleanor Noss Whitney. *Nutrition: Concepts and Controversies.* 12th edition. Wadsworth, Cengage Learning, 2011.

Articles:

1. 4-Mozaffarian D et al. PLoS med 201023: 7 e10000252 Meta-Analysis of Randomized Controlled Trials-Displacing with PUFA, Carbohydate, MUFA

2. Am J Clin Nutr. 2010 Mar;91(3):502-9. Epub 2010 Jan 20.
    Saturated fat, carbohydrate, and cardiovascular disease.
    Siri-Tarino PW, Sun Q, Hu FB, Krauss RM.

3. Cochrane Database Update
    WITHDRAWN: Advice on low-fat diets for obesity.

    Summerbell CD, Cameron C, Glasziou PP.

4. Regular egg consumption does not increase the risk of stroke and cardiovascular diseases.

    Qureshi AI, Suri FK, Ahmed S, Nasar A, Divani AA, Kirmani JF.

    Epub 2011 Jan 26.
    Astrup A Dyerberg J, Elwood P, Hermansen K, Hu FB, Jakobsen MU, Kok FJ, Krauss RM, Lecerf JM, LeGrand P, Nestel P, Risérus U, Sanders T, Sinclair A, Stender S, Tholstrup T, Willett WC.

The role of reducing intakes of saturated fat in the prevention of cardiovascular disease: where does the evidence stand in 2010?
"Furthermore, the effect of particular foods on CHD cannot be predicted solely by their content of total SFAs because individual SFAs may have different cardiovascular effects and major SFA food sources contain other constituents that could influence CHD risk."

Epub 2010 Jan 20.
Saturated fat, carbohydrate, and cardiovascular disease.
Siri-Tarino PW, Sun Q, Hu FB, Krauss RM.
"An independent association of saturated fat intake with CVD risk has not been consistently shown in prospective epidemiologic studies, although some have provided evidence of an increased risk in young individuals and in women."

Epub 2010 Mar 31.
Saturated fat and cardiometabolic risk factors, coronary heart disease, stroke, and diabetes: a fresh look at the evidence.
Micha R, Mozaffarian D.
"Compared with carbohydrate, the TC:HDL-C ratio is nonsignificantly affected by consumption of myristic or palmitic acid, is nonsignificantly decreased by stearic acid, and is significantly decreased by lauric acid."

"Evidence for the effects of SFA consumption on vascular function, insulin resistance, diabetes, and stroke is mixed, with many studies showing no clear effects."

Index

A

ABPS (Association of Bariatric Physicians), 123–24
adipocytes, 7–8, 26, 67, 226, 244, 248, 259, 261, 286
AIM-HIGH trial, 5
antioxidants, 27, 46, 79, 232, 262, 264
apple obesity, 6, 17, 125, 128
Aronne, Louis J., 25–26, 133, 258, 295
  Skinny, The, 25–26, 137, 258, 295
Ash, Arthur, 32
Atkins, Robert, 226–27
Atkins diet, 58, 123, 227, 238, 250–51
A-Z trial, 58, 123, 127, 238, 251, 253, 264, 268

B

Bailar, John, 288
Bell, John Steward, 274
Bishops Palace. *See* Wurzburg Residence
Bouchard, Claude, 40, 133, 138

Bray, George, 20, 67, 72, 223, 286
  Guide to Obesity and the Metabolic Syndrome, A, 67, 72, 223, 234, 255, 286, 295
Brillat-Savarin, 223
Brody, Jane, 228
Burch, Hilde, 224
Burma, 42, 85, 158

C

Caballero, Benjamin, 56, 59, 136
Cahill, George, 226
Cain, Herman, 13
carbohydrates, 24, 26, 86, 128, 226, 264
comparative diet trial, 58, 123, 145, 238, 264
Cooper, Ken, 133
Cruise, Jorge, 18, 25, 123, 129

D

Dancel, Francois, 224
Dr. Spock, 225
Dr. Superko, 36

E

EE (energy expenditure), 15, 68, 232, 236

F

fat cells. *See* adipocytes
Fat Head, 68, 124, 246
Fen-phen, 270
Fixx, Jim, 32, 133
food religion, 46
Framingham score, 36

G

Gauguin, Paul, 77–79, 91–92, 221
ghrelin, 16, 130, 258
Gordon, Edgar, 226
Gordon, Jeffrey, 131
Greene, Raymond, 225
Guide to Obesity and the Metabolic Syndrome, A (Bray), 67, 72, 223, 234, 255, 286, 295
gut microbes, 67, 259

H

Hall of Mirrors, 89
Harvey, William, 224
Hawaii, 3, 49–50, 57, 79, 88, 91, 165
HDL, 27, 37–38, 63, 124–25
Heindel, Jerry, 131
Hill, H. Gardiner, 225
Hirsch, Jules, 137, 244, 254
Hong Kong, 36, 41–42, 47, 85–86, 214

I

India, 2, 43, 86, 159, 175, 220
insulin, 24, 26, 46, 226, 228
insulin resistance, 227, 259–60, 265
Interleukin Genetics Inc., 131

K

Kendrick, Malcolm, 69, 246–47
Keys, Ancel, 15, 69, 137, 227, 237, 244–45
Kolata, Gina, 40, 59, 132, 135–38, 222, 248
    Rethinking Thin, 56, 59, 135–37, 222, 244, 248, 254, 295
    Ultimate Fitness, 40, 132–33, 138, 258, 295
Kris-Etherton, Penny, 122

L

Lasker, Mary, 288
leptin, 67–68
leptin resistance, 8, 13, 26, 259
leptin threshold, 7–8, 13, 15, 67–68, 231, 236, 254, 259, 264, 270
lipidology, 5, 13, 16
Look AHEAD trial, 255

M

Mayer, Jean, 227, 238, 242
metabolic syndrome, 43, 46, 59, 64, 86, 125, 128, 134, 227, 232, 263–65
metformin, 36–37, 47, 58, 82, 124, 129
Moore, Jimmy, 69, 246
Mr. Banting, 224
Mukherjee, Siddhartha, 287, 289
Myanmar, 2, 42, 85

N

Naughton, Tom, 124
NEJM (*New England Journal of Medicine*), 124, 130, 135, 251, 288
NLa (National Lipidology association), 36, 46, 85, 123–24, 128, 138, 288
Non-HDL cholesterol, 6, 10, 15, 27, 37, 245, 283
nutrition science, 124

O

obesity, 32, 34, 43, 58, 66, 76, 140, 223, 225–26, 256, 258–61
Obesity Society, 13, 67–68, 91, 123, 128, 235
Ornish, 37, 124, 145, 232–33, 238, 249–51
Osler, William, 224

P

Pennington, Alfred, 225
Peripheral fat, 62

R

reduced obese, 6, 13–18, 59, 66–68, 79–80, 126, 232, 235–36, 244, 246, 256–57, 259, 265
Rethinking Thin (Kolata), 59, 135–37, 222, 248, 254, 295
Russert, Tim, 69

S

Sachs, Frank, 20, 58, 232, 264, 268
Schindler, Oskar, 89
Sheehan, George, 133
Shwedagon Pagoda, 85
Sims, Ethan, 137, 248, 254
Singapore, 2, 42, 85, 157
Sistine Chapel, 89
Skinny, The (Aronne), 25–26, 137, 258, 295
Smith, Elaine, 288
Sniderman, Allan, 69
Sponge Syndrome, 8, 12–15, 18, 59, 66, 68, 123, 125, 128–30, 134, 140, 231, 236, 256, 291
statin, 10, 27, 69, 241, 246–47, 277, 282, 288–89, 292
Stunkard, Mickey, 44, 144, 222
Stunkark, Albert J., 134

T

Tanner, Thomas, 224
Taubes, Gary, 24, 26, 36, 47, 124, 129, 223, 226–29, 232, 238
    Why We Get Fat, 24, 26, 36, 47, 124, 223, 232, 238
thailand, 2, 42, 85, 156, 218
Thorpe, George, 225
three-hour diet, 18, 25, 123, 129
Tiepolo, G. B., 89

U

Ultimate Fitness (Kolata), 40, 132–33, 138, 258, 295

V

VaP, 27, 37, 63–64, 125
Vietnam, 2, 42, 85

W

weight loss, 26–27
Westman, Eric, 88
Why We Get Fat (Taubes), 24, 26, 36, 47, 124, 223, 232, 238
Willett, Walter C., 122, 241
Wittgenstein, 135
Wurzburg residence, 89

Y

Young, Charlotte, 226

CPSIA information can be obtained at www.ICGtesting.com
Printed in the USA
LVOW111951081012

302049LV00002B/1/P